LOVING

YOU

THROUGH

IT

An Image of Sisterhood

Copyright © 2018 by Misha Stredrick

LOVING YOU THROUGH IT

An Image of Sisterhood

Misha Stredrick

Contents

For my mother, Carla May, and the women in my family...love you, Mimi.

ACKNOWLEDGMENTS

Thank you, God, for allowing Your thoughts to translate to my paper and for trusting me with this task!

To my family, thank you for loving and supporting me through every turn that God has allowed me to experience. Each trial, decision, and success has led me to this very moment. I'm proud to share it with you, especially my mother and father, Carla and Derrick Stredrick!

Thank you to every woman who has contributed to my growth and became a guide in my life. To my grandmothers, Mrs. Woods, and the late Mrs. Wright, and unofficial church mothers, who had a hand in keeping me on track as a child: Mrs. Reynolds, Mrs. English, Mrs. Black, Mrs. McWilson, and the two Mrs. Catherines, you are/were the women I watched and mimicked. Thank you for being such great examples. To the first ladies, Mrs. Small, Mrs. McBee, and Mrs. Heard, thank you for helping me to understand the contrast between womanhood and spirituality. To Mrs. Allen, Mrs. Baldwin, and Ms. Seimetz, thank you for being authentic at all times...love you all! To my spiritual advisors, Pastor Heard and Pastor Walker, words cannot express what your support means. Thank you for following the heart of God and steering me in the direction of holiness, even when I wanted to veer off!

Thank you to each friend and family member who tolerated my interviews, questions, and illogical ramblings. LaQuesha Stredrick, Michelle Curry, Crystal Kramer, Maria Diaz, LaDonna Newell, Stacy Warfield, Summer Carter, Dovonna Smith, Eboni Williams, Christina Scissum, Darla Jones, Jennifer Andes, Tanera Graham, Quiana Faison, Kim Lawrence, Montez Lockett, and Robin Wesson, thank you for your honesty, vulnerability, and patience.

To my spiritual mother, Co-Pastor Kim Walker, you have helped me transition naturally and spiritually. It is not often that you run into someone whose character is matched perfectly with her spiritual purpose. God knew exactly what He was doing when He placed you in my journey!

To Andrell Williams, David Turner and Michael Reynolds, for conveying my message and vision into this finished product…THANK YOU! I pray God opens unimaginable doors for you!

Thank YOU for supporting this book. I pray it leads you to examine the women around you and/or challenges you to become better women, individually and collectively. My prayer is for us all to become who God intended us to be!

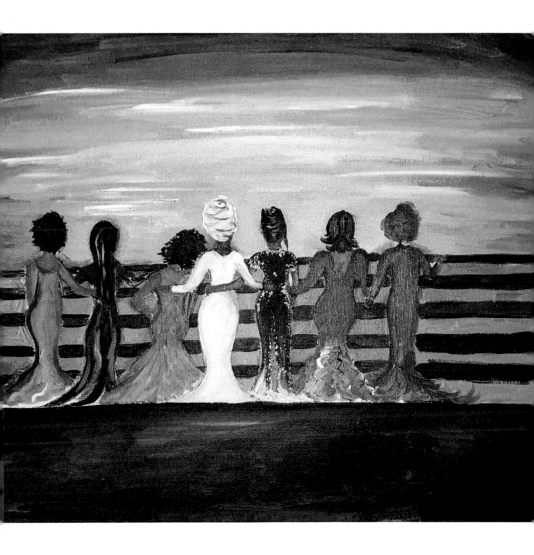

FOREWORD

I remember the day I met Misha Stredrick. I walked into the adult Sunday school class at Restoration Christian Fellowship Church and sat in the back of the sanctuary, as the class was already in session. As I looked around observing those in attendance and listening to their responses to the questions presented by the teacher, my eyes fell upon a young lady sitting several rows in front of me whom I had never seen before. While it was not uncommon for visitors and guests to attend the Sunday school class from time to time, there was something very different about this young lady that caught my eye and commanded my attention. Her body language spoke volumes of her eager pursuit of God. Practically sitting on the edge of her seat listening as the teacher instructed, it was apparent that she panted after God as the deer pants after the water brooks, and as she raised her hand and began to speak, I knew I had come in contact with one whose heart's language I understood and whose passion for a deeper level of intimacy with God I shared.

Little did I know that from that moment on this spiritual connection would evolve into one of trust, support, encouragement, honesty, wise counsel, and genuine friendship. Little did I know that that this young lady, who was about to experience a whirlwind of devastating and painful events in her life, would become a spiritual daughter to my husband and me, and that the next two years of my life would be spent journeying with her through the lowlands to the high places as part of her spiritual support team.

Within months of our first encounter, not only had Misha become an active member of our church, but God had navigated my career path right to the doorstep of the place where she spent well over forty hours each week. The job I applied for, before I ever knew Misha's occupation, led me to an assignment in the building in which she served as principal. God knit our lives together in a very unique way. I knew that God had placed me in her life much like He places a midwife in the life of a woman preparing to give birth. There were gifts within Misha that needed to come forth. There was a calling upon her life that needed to be revealed. However, not without pain, not without discomfort, not without testing, and not without trials, and the more she suffered, the more she sought God. The more she experienced brokenness and despair, the more she pressed into God's presence. The more she suffered humiliation, the more she humbled herself and rested under the mighty hand of God, knowing that He would, in due season, exalt her.

On her journey to the high places, I saw Misha count the cost and daily renew her mind through reading and studying God's Word and speaking His Word over her life. She built her spiritual muscles by walking by faith and exercising the spiritual gifts God placed within her. She made fasting and prayer a significant part of her daily life, and she sought the face of God continually to make sure she did not lose ground despite the strong winds she encountered along the way. The more she sought God, the more He revealed Himself, and the more He revealed Himself, the more she sought Him. Not only did God heal her, but He loved her into wholeness. He was her oxygen, He was her peace. He taught her to trust Him. He taught her to believe beyond what she could see.

It is my prayer that as you read this book, you will gain a deeper understanding of God's amazing love for you. Despite the many difficult challenges that we face in life, God is faithful to meet our needs and to love us through every hard place. "The LORD is like a father to his children, tender and compassionate to those who fear him. For he knows how weak we are; he remembers we are only dust. But the love of the LORD remains forever…" (Psalm 103:13–14, 17a

NLT). May this book serve as a source of inspiration, impartation, and transformation as you make your ascent to the high places.

Kimberly D. Walker

Co-Pastor, Restoration Christian Fellowship Church

UNPACKING MY SUITCASE

Allow me to be vulnerable for a moment, as I give you the details that led me to the vision of this book. No ordinary circumstances could have resulted in finding out that the most important relationships I would encounter as a woman were with other women. I know that sounds like a normal concept, but when you have lived a life where you have convinced yourself that men were easier to deal with, this concept is anything but normal. In fact, it is foreign!

If anyone told me that I would encounter something so traumatic it would cause me to lean on and trust women significantly, I would have said they were tripping. Then it happened! I smile thinking about God's strategy to place me in a situation that would force me to examine the nature of Christian sisterhood. I'm sure He knew that I would be amazed at the relationships with women I needed during this time. I cultivated priceless friendships when I needed wisdom, comfort, love, understanding, nurturing, and compassion. I needed someone to talk to and walk this journey out with, while my heart was being lifted.

Have you ever been there?

In a place where you just needed to know that someone cared?

There I was. I needed someone who understood my struggle and would help me unpack my emotions. So God surrounded me with supportive women who connected me to God's purpose for my life. It was a setup! God wanted me to experience the power that manifests when women come together and unite with a real purpose. This truth is the premise of this book.

I intend for you to reflect on the women who have challenged you to LOVE THROUGH and who were challenged to LOVE YOU

THROUGH IT. These women loved you through hurt, pain, struggles, confusion, and unbelief. They were vital to your growth and assisted you with life's transitions. This book is a reflection of these women. The women who made my life easier, helped me believe, and reminded me that I was loved. They surrounded me with love while I was discovering a new version of myself. They made my journey manageable and helped me regain composure with their examples of strength, hope, and vulnerability. And they did it while representing God!

I challenge you to read this book and identify with each woman. Ask yourself: Who is this type of sister? Do I know someone like her? Do I have her characteristics? And does she bring value to the Kingdom of God? Reflect throughout the pages, review each sister's character, and complete the tasks, by yourself or with a friend. Grow as you recognize that God can speak through women about purpose and determination. And challenge yourself to look at which women in your life are LOVING YOU THROUGH IT...

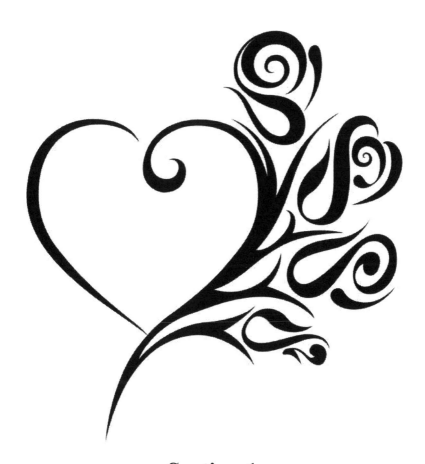

Section 1

LIVE WITH EASE

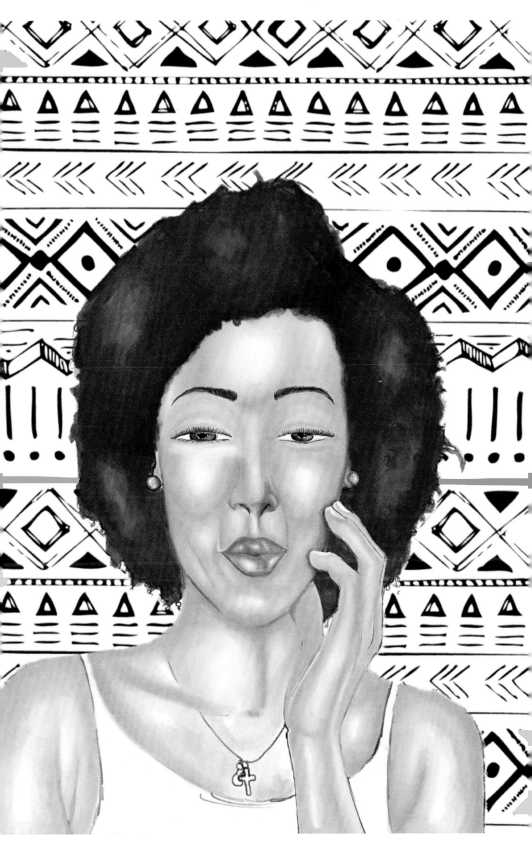

THE AIR I BREATHE

The air I breathe now standing atop the mountain. Looking down on the path that I took.

Rewarding.

How it knocked the wind out of me at different turns

Life was a head blow with an uppercut.

No amount of covering could protect my mind from the set that left me staggering.

Reaching for the ropes to hold on to

I spit at the thought that my opponents would very well be those who made vows to protect me and coach me through life.

Through sickness and in health. Till death do you part.

Now I stand at the coffin.

Breathing deeply.

Holding back a wail inside that would upset and awaken those sleeping in deep graves.

I isolated myself

So my breath would not contaminate the already polluted mentality

They have me messed up!

But I exhale

While lying at the feet of God. His altar provided protection.

Directions.

A constant in this variable circumstance.

A space where my breathing matched God's heartbeat

For the first time in forever, I was aligned with no interference

In alignment without dragging the weight of another.

His weight was no longer my weight, and I began to soar to a new altitude.

Taking in all that surrounded me. I walked when God said walk. Ran when God said run.

Inhaling the fragrance that was pleasing to God.

Obedience became my daily bread.

And it fed my desire to sync my movement with the hand of God.

I gave up the ghost to reach forward. My unknown destiny.

Each stretch of faith is like a puff of inhalation. It revives my ability to breathe.

Once completely asphyxiated with the lack, I now experience what it feels to catch my breath.

puff...Release the pain. *puff*...Release poverty. *puff*...Release sadness.

puff...Release anger. *puff*...Release confusion. *puff*...Release hate.

God breathed into my being like Adam's lifeless body, and I was immediately

Made whole.

He that believeth shall have an everlasting life

I believe in the wind of God

And my deliverance

I now see the importance of my breathing.

This is the air I breathe.

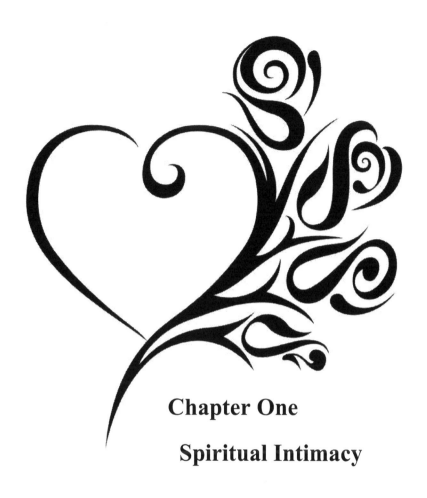

Chapter One

Spiritual Intimacy

"A PERSONAL JOURNEY"

SPIRITUAL AWAKENING

Here I am. Living in a very complex moment and experiencing one of the most significant transitions in my life. My job is terrible, my health is failing, my marriage is falling apart, multiple people are plotting against me…and God has the nerve to have me learning about my spiritual gifts. How could He possibly think this is the time? I've been living as if life were grand, but right now my mental space is horrible and I feel as if I'm losing it! I'm drained and no longer wish to live this way. This season has brought me to the point where I cannot continue like this. This day, I had to make a choice:

Continue to deny that I need help.

Or ask God what I need to do and surrender.

One would think this would be a simple decision, but I began to consider the options. How far in denial was I? What would surrendering mean for me? And how would either decision impact my lifestyle? I was inquisitive about the consequences that chasing the wrong choice would bring. It didn't take long before I admitted I needed the change. Surrendering was the answer! However, I needed God to help me with trusting Him. I needed Him to give me references for how to allow Him to lead. I needed to be honest, I had no idea how "surrendering" was supposed to go.

"Yea, though I walk through the valley of the shadow of death, I will fear no evil: for thou art with me; thy rod and thy staff they comfort me." (Psalm 23:4 KJV)

I felt like this dramatic scripture was my life. I WAS walking through the valley of the shadow of death. There, everything around me looked like it was dying. I saw bleakness in my personal and professional life; yet I knew in my heart I was not called to be afraid. God did not intend for me to stop moving. Instead, He wanted me to be confident. I admit, I often asked Him how He could expect me to be confident when I had no frame of reference for what was occurring. This valley was calling for me to yell out, "I will fear no evil," but the attacks didn't stop. God wanted me to look around and recognize the evil looks, the mean words, the slander, and the lies, and still declare, "I will fear no evil." I had become so comfortable looking at my situations that God now required me to change my mind-set. Instead of living in the "valley of the shadow of death," God asked me to speak over the "dying" things I was walking through.

Have you ever been there?

In a place where God is telling you to relinquish all efforts while demanding you to speak over your circumstances?

If you have, you know this is not a comfortable place. It goes against everything you are taught and requires you to speak about things that are not visible like they are already happening. Talk about strange…

"…and calleth those things which be not as though they were." *(Romans 4:17 KJV)*

This foreign concept is a newfound place of spiritual freedom that forces you to leave your own visual senses and depend on God for insight. You must dismiss what you see and believe that whatever God has spoken has already manifested. I know this sounds crazy, but you can deny what you see in the natural. Let me give you an example:

Each morning when I awake, I make the assumption that there will still be clothes in my closet. I have no idea what I am going to wear…but I am confident that the outfit exists. I will pass up multiple articles of clothing, confident that "the one" will stand out to me. This process can take anywhere from five minutes to two hours; however, when an outfit finally speaks to me, I feel a sense of relief because I knew this outfit was there all along. Just as confident as I am that this outfit exists, God is calling me to be this confident when it comes to everything else! Even when I don't immediately see it, my belief should stay intact as I search for it. How often do you actively search for what God has promised? Or speak about the promise like it has manifested itself? Surrendering to God calls for us to enter a different level of freedom, and the first step is to "call things which are not as though they were." Instead of worrying about your situation, God is telling you to stop looking at what you see and focus on what you see in your spirit. This is what I refer to as your spiritual eyes. Your spiritual eyes allow you to tap into what God has spoken versus what you see in the natural.

- Yes, in the natural my job was a wreck, but I needed to see myself spiritually in a position that brings joy and allows me to excel to another level.
- Yes, in the natural my heart was broken, but I needed to see myself spiritually whole and healed from the pain.
- Yes, in the natural my life seemed to be falling apart, but I needed to see myself in a state of wholeness.
- Yes, in the natural my emotions were all out of control, but I needed to see myself spiritually showcasing an excellent level of self-control and confidence.

To begin this season, God needed me to practice being in sync with Him. I needed to exert my effort in believing that God was going to use this valley to catapult me into a new way of life. And God started by giving me His first three spiritual applications of purpose...

Spiritual Application of Purpose #1:

Speak What You Do Not See as if You Already Have It

- Just because it has not come to fruition does not mean it will never happen.
- Keep speaking it! If you are in alignment with God, you can speak things into existence.

Spiritual Application of Purpose #2:

If What You Speak Is Not Occurring, Actively Seek God in Prayer to Ensure That What You Are Speaking Is in God's Will

- Prayer and communication with God will allow you access to God's heart concerning what you are seeking.
- Be mindful that God will never give you something that goes against His Word. Example: You are not in God's will if you are asking God to give you someone else's husband. You may be functioning in a spirit of lust or envy, but you are definitely not in God's will.

Spiritual Application of Purpose #3:

Learn How God Speaks to You

- Take a moment to ask God about one circumstance in your life.

- Pray for God to release all unnecessary thoughts from your mind, especially the ones that are unlike God, and ask God to speak to you about that circumstance.
- Sit, in absolute silence, and write down what you hear in your spirit.

DRAWING CLOSER TO GOD

God's plan is for us to learn how to align with Him, listen for His guidance, and believe that we have power. But what do you do when you are struggling with this? When I began this journey, my heart was set on finding the answer to the question "Why?" Why am I in this season? Why can't I know what will occur in the future? By asking too many questions that began with "why," I was saying that these answers were more important than the act of listening to God. Anyone could ask questions, but God was asking me to add the concept of "actively hearing what God is speaking over my life," to "speaking things as though they were." God was asking me to hear with my spiritual ears.

Much like speaking, using your spiritual ears will require you to regularly ingest scripture and be strategic about how you connect with God. This is necessary so you can decipher what God is speaking to you. While seeking Him, will you need to know what God says about marriage? About friendships? About betrayal? About being broken? About our Christian walk? You will need to become relentless in your pursuit of God and be intentional about what you are seeking Him for. This was the place where I began to embrace the purpose that God was leading me to. I had determined that although my natural ears were hearing failure, my spiritual ears were hearing "I can do all things through Christ which strengthened me" (Philippians 4:13 KJV). And although my natural ears were hearing "I do not have the energy to fight," my spiritual ears were hearing "the Lord who rescued me from the paw of the lion and the paw of the bear will rescue me from the hand of this Philistine." (1 Samuel 17:37 NIV). Hearing what God was saying in this challenging season was what led me to victories. For God to grow me, I needed to take time to hear from Him and follow the directions He was sending me.

THE PERSONAL EXAMINATION

Moving forward, I began to ask myself, "What kind of woman am I?" I had to take a long look in the mirror and identify the woman I had become. Not just the woman in the struggle, but the conglomerate of my past and current experiences...who have they created? I began to examine all facets of me...spiritually, physically, and emotionally. I had to recognize that I was becoming more intimate with God, and it was opening a personal awareness that I had never experienced! In this time period, I was becoming very clear about the fact that I was lost. I had never acknowledged it before, but God was revealing that I had been slowly giving away myself to become someone else. This new person was someone between who the world needed and who I thought I should be. God was making it very clear that I was more concerned about everyone else than I was with God. So now I needed to ask, "Who does God need me to be?" Because it was clear that not asking Him had led me to a place where I didn't even recognize myself!

Have you ever been there?

In a place where you are working hard to become someone that you know you are not?

On the outside, you seem stronger than ever; yet inwardly, you are imploding. You are not growing and nothing is feeding your spirit, but you are too afraid to let people know. You're considering the question, "What would they do if they knew I was dying here?" There I was. Perfecting crafts that were not beneficial to me and staying stagnant to appease those around me. I wanted more out of life. More than encouraging others to break free and believe in themselves. I needed to break free myself! I was living in turmoil, knowing that this life equated misery to me. Small thoughts and ideas, disbelief that God could do abundant things... How did I end up in a place where I was settling? I became the load bearer for many, but I recognized that my most massive load was not living up to my own potential.

So I repented for hearing God but not following Him, and I surrendered my life to Him again. This time I prayed specific prayers of peace, spiritual growth, personal growth, deliverance, and for God to reign over everything in my life. As God began to work in my heart, I was starting to understand that surrendering was requiring me to give up everything. Everything! I had to release shame, pain, embarrassment, and every question I had and was waiting for God to answer. At that moment, I asked God about marriage, my family, my job, my ministry, and even His opinion on who I needed to become.

I poured out my heart and took pride in knowing that God was listening. Then He asked me, "Who do you think you are?" This was a great question because, at this very moment, I had no idea! The personal and spiritual inconsistencies within my life had made this question difficult to answer. I mean, I could say I believed I was more than a conqueror, but I often acted defeated. I could say I can do all things through Christ who strengthens me, but I often discovered a weak mentality. I could say that I was the head and not the tail, but my crawling and limping around made me closer to the ground than to the sky. Finally, after taking a long look at myself, I was able to admit...I was a woman who was wounded. It took the life out of me to say it, but it was true. Yes, I was a soldier for Christ, but I was definitely not equipped for fighting anything right now. I needed Jesus to nurse me back to health. Spiritually, emotionally, and physically. I needed to be healthy again. I believe this is the reason why God allowed things to shake up in my life...He heard the prayers

I made and knew to get where He wanted me to be, I would have to start anew. This newer version of me would have a different narrative. I was no longer able to live in the monotony of my past life, God was calling me to a higher place. I knew this but had no idea what that place was.

Have you ever been there?

In a place where you no longer fit the mold of the past, but you are not quite in the new season?

There I was! Living beyond the catastrophe but waiting on the catalyst for my increase. I knew God was grooming me for something amazing. It had to be the reason why He allowed me to endure so much pain. I was destined for something, and the previous season was helping me move toward it. I felt like this level of attack in my life meant that God intended me to become fluent in the tricks of the enemy. For some reason, I would need to have this experience to share with someone else; but today, I needed the help! I needed His Word to feed my spirit. I needed people who could physically walk this journey with me. I needed new relationships that would help my spiritual intimacy with God. And I needed these relationships to be pleasing to God. This led me to inspect my surroundings. Who were the people around me? Were they able to help me become who God intended me to be? Were they working on themselves in a manner that would please God? Were they accountable for living their lives in a godly way, or were they just living haphazardly? Did I respect their walk with Christ enough to allow them to hold me accountable? Was I able to hold them accountable? I knew that this upcoming season would require a different level of friendships...specifically, a different level of sisterhood.

I would need wise women around me who were responsible, accountable, encouraging, and discerning. I needed them to see when

I could not and hear when I refused. This was when God gave me the six women you will read of in this book.

1. The faithful sister
2. The struggling sister
3. The sister with trust issues
4. The sister who is a mentor
5. The sister who opens opportunities
6. The sister who is a spiritual mother

Each of these women helped me to transition from a place of stagnation to a place where God is allowing me to blossom into who He wants me to be. These women gave me the viewpoints of God without judgment while I experienced the struggle. They held my hand and bent their ears as I grew. They took my walk with Christ seriously. They listened as I cried, they pushed when I hesitated, and they prayed when I was uncertain. They helped me to get through a painful season and prayed me through to the other side. I needed all of them. Collectively and individually, I needed them. They remained true to themselves while making a way for me to be honest about who I was. These women held me accountable to God's Word, even when straying from it would be more comfortable. They served as my cheerleaders and my examples of strength in God. I was able to use their viewpoints to grow into my next level of intimacy with God. It is my prayer that you recognize yourself and the women around you within these chapters describing each woman.

MAY YOU "LOVE THROUGH" THESE QUESTIONS:

- Which sister types do you believe you have around you? The faithful sister, the struggling sister, the sister with trust issues, the sister who is a mentor, the sister who opens opportunities, or the sister who is a spiritual mother?

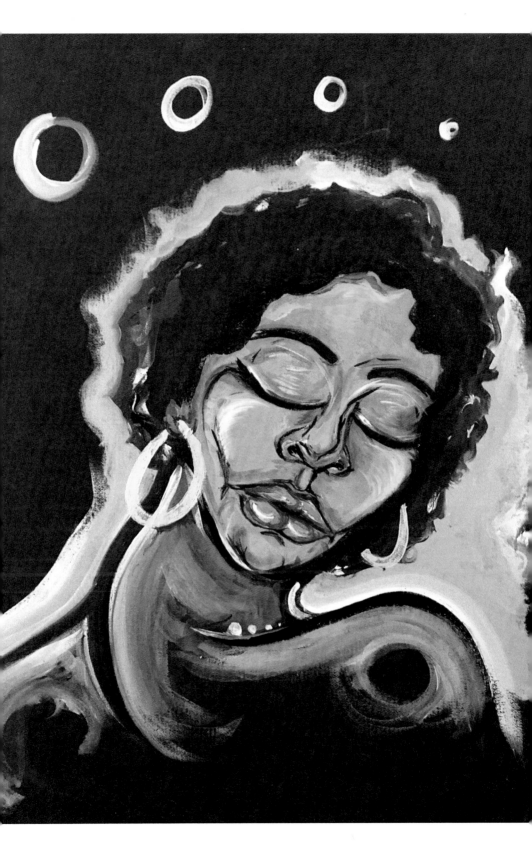

TIMELESS FRIENDSHIP

Get you one!

A friend so close to your heart that speaking to her feels like home

A planet-shaking friendship that will outlast all phases of life

From glory to glory

It remains.

An ageless truth that withstands the test of time but does not go untested

These tests come outwardly, yet also dwell within

What do you do when she questions your motives? Or your desires?

How do you stand up to confrontation when you know inwardly you are out of bounds?

She calls you out

Constantly reminding you as to who you were

Where you are going

And what you need to do to get there

She gets it!

In a trying-your-soul, while-tiring-out-your-mind kind of way

She wants you to succeed

While acknowledging her own struggle

Girl, I can't lie…she shouts as you reveal your flaws one by one

She is Help.

Although you're not quite helpless, you require a different type of support

A gentle push.

A stern look.

And a punch to the gut. Every now and then

You need it and she gives it.

Connecting herself to your God and recalibrating her moods, actions, and emotions

She wants to be aligned.

She wants you to be aligned.

She helps you to be consistent in your momentum for Christ.

For your walk is equally important...you have a grand purpose

And she knows it.

Owns it.

Points you to it.

Get you one!

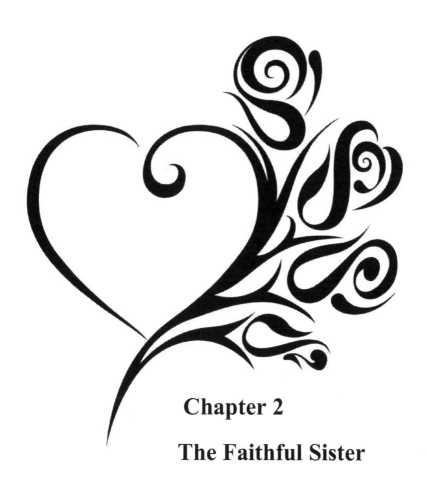

Chapter 2

The Faithful Sister

TECHNICAL ASSISTANCE

ALLIES

I sit and observe her going through a variety of emotions. My sister. I am the connection between her feelings and our God today. As she expresses her hurt and anguish, it is my responsibility to filter through and channel it. She goes off, and I let her; I help her process. Although I admit that sometimes it's hard not to go off with her, but today I am trying. I am trying to ride through every wave of life with her. The good, the bad, the ugly, and the glorious. I take the concept of this seriously. Living for seeing her growth in Christ, while recognizing the need for all old ways and habits to die. I love our conversations of comparison! She reminds me where I've come from, and I recall the same for her. Any characteristic unlike God that remains has to go. We are preparing ourselves for greater things!

Today was unlike our usual conversations. I recognized the tone of a crisis in my sister's voice. She sounds like she's in a dark place. Not clearly seeing it herself, but I realize it. Defeat and darkness have surrounded her, and I listen as she tries to fight this feeling. Praying about what God needs me to do. Does He want me to strictly be a listener today? Or is He going to permit me the ability to speak? Invitation or not, I intend to come through with an encouraging word for her. I need to be in alignment with what God requires. I care too much about her to steer her in a wrong direction and too much about God to go against what He desires. So I watch and wait for a moment to speak.

"Let every man be swift to hear, slow to speak..." (James 1:19 KJV)

While I pray for her, I pray for myself as well. I know I should be focused entirely on her, but I need God to check me. I desired Him to put to death my sharp tongue and aggressive behavior, as I awaited His instructions. *Take me out of the equation. Allow my flesh to die so*

I can encourage her spirit. I had to ask God to impart wisdom while I tune in to her story. I need guidance on what to do. I need to be spiritually ready to prepare her to keep believing. I have her back because I know today is her day, but tomorrow may be my day of crisis. The future may hold many days when I need elevated faith, but today she needs me to step outside my comfort zone and be the rock for her.

Have you ever been there?

In a place where God is expecting you to hold off your issues and exhibit your strength for others?

There I was. Interacting with my sister yet called to showcase a strength that I didn't even know I had. God was calling me to show her how not to be offended and lose self-control when in reality I wanted to scream myself. I had to point out the discrepancies without being offended when her words had the potential to cut me like a knife. I had to be transparent and vulnerable. Sharing statements that would help her to gain sight of God while helping me to maintain my spiritual freedom. Who told God that I could be this accountable? Even if this level of accountability provided peace and healing to both of us, it was going to be a constant personal struggle. One that admiration couldn't get me through. This time I had to be raw...really raw. This conversation would entail more than "How are you doing?" It would discuss the question "How is your spirit?" It would address the topic of healing and peeling back layers of her heart. This type of intimate conversation will soon become the staple of our friendship.

Spiritual Application of Purpose #4:

Make Intimate Conversations a Norm

- Analyze how many transparent conversations you have had with sisters.

48

- Ask yourself the following questions: Can I be vulnerable enough to express my flaws, weaknesses, and secrets to them? Can they do the same?
- Are you sure that your friends will give you a position that aligns with what God says and thinks?

TRAIN WITH ME

Our friendship is a place of vulnerability. A place where we share as much as we listen. Opening our hearts, while acknowledging our flaws. This journey is requiring us both to gain freedom with each other by speaking openly about everything. However, this takes time and trust. My sisters are like gym partners for my soul. We become dedicated to seeing each other accomplish the task. Both spiritually and personally, we set goals to work on and track each other crushing them.

"No, dear brothers and sisters, I have not achieved it, but I focus on this one thing: Forgetting the past and looking forward to what lies ahead. I press on to reach the end of the race and receive the heavenly prize for which God, through Christ Jesus, is calling us."

(Philippians 3:13–14 NLT)

Training beside my sister requires me to be humble and reflective. "I count not myself to have apprehended," translates to admittedly not achieving the mark; while "pressing towards the mark," acknowledges that I still have work to do. Goals become a staple of our friendship and it doesn't matter if our goal is the same. All that matters is that we show up and train. We are preparing to do the work that God has placed inside of us. This will be hard work!

The work of sharing the unfinished parts of your spirit means you must search through your own heart and expose who you are. We all can give feedback and coach when needed, but what occurs when you must push through who you are? I must exude a consistent light for my sister. Through dark moments, I need her to see the real me, just as much as she needs me to see the real her. I need her to understand that "I'm struggling today," without hearing the words. The training of sisterhood has allowed us to relate, shed tears, and initiate coaching sessions. So the question "How is your spirit?" remained.

Not every conversation is this serious, but we have learned not to mince words about God's purpose. I laugh thinking about how the most straightforward topic can lead back to God's will. Taking out the trash can turn into a natural example of how God intends for us to rid or reuse situations in our lives. Choice of foods can turn into discussions about the spiritual food we eat and how over time your palate should become more refined. I love our conversations! Hearty laughs, unforgettable scenarios, and challenges to my heart are what I look forward to each time. I am challenged and refreshed in every dialogue. When I am wrong, she checks me. When she is out of order, I check her and hold her to a godly standard. Women of Christ should have other women helping them to meet the expectation.

DON'T GIVE UP

Don't fret if you have not attained this level of sisterhood; it means you and your friends have work to do. Your work will require you to address your level of intimacy. Can you genuinely handle someone having access to your heart? I'm not referring to your likes and dislikes, I'm referring to the reasons behind them. The secrets that you haven't shared with anyone. Which sisters genuinely know the intimate details of your heart? The stories that you are ashamed to say aloud and the moments you regret...who knows those stories? Sharing these parts of our testimonies are not just for the telling of your story, but to bring revelation to the elements of your life that God is trying to grow. Have you allowed God to examine your heart?

The work of your sisters is a little more straightforward. You must ask God to reveal which friendships are Christ-led. It will be easy to recognize these friendships, as they will always challenge your thinking with God's truth.

If you're a fornicator, they will talk to you about your body being a temple for the Holy Spirit.

"Don't you realize that your body is the temple of the Holy Spirit, who lives in you and was given to you by God? You do not belong to yourself." (1 Corinthians 6:19 NLT)

If you are a gossiper, they will talk to you about speaking the truth from a sincere heart and not harming neighbors.

"Who may worship in your sanctuary, LORD? Who may enter your presence on your holy hill? Those who lead blameless lives and do what is right, speaking truth from sincere hearts. Those who refuse to gossip or harm their neighbors or speak evil of their friends." (Psalm 15:1–3 NLT)

If you are an adulterer, they will talk to you about the marital covenant being a natural illustration of your relationship with and respect for God.

"And further, submit to one another out of reverence for Christ." (Ephesians 5:21 NLT)

If you harbor hatred in your heart, they will talk to you about how everything you do means nothing without love.

"If I had the gift of prophecy, and if I understood all of God's secret plans and possessed all knowledge, and if I had such faith that I could move mountains, but didn't love others, I would be nothing. If I gave everything I have to the poor and even sacrificed my body, I could boast about it; but if I didn't love others, I would have gained nothing." (1 Corinthians 13:2–3 NLT)

This type of friend is hard to be around; yet it is refreshing knowing you don't have to hide any part of you. To come by a sister like this, you may have to relieve superficial friends from your circle. If your sister isn't correcting your ungodly ways, then she is probably not equipped to be a "faithful" sister.

SHE BRINGS EASE

It is imperative that this type of sisterhood comes with an initial fight that eventually leads to an easiness. It's not easy being an accountability partner who fights for someone else's life! A sister knows what she will say may not be popular, but it will need to be told. I have been that sister. And I have needed that sister!

For me to grow into the woman God was calling me to be, I needed the honesty of someone who had my best interests at heart. I needed the compassion of someone who understood my sentiments and the reliability of someone who would still love me, in spite of my decisions…I needed that sister. I am that sister!

MAY YOU "LOVE THROUGH" THESE QUESTIONS:

COULD YOU BE HER? The "Faithful Sister"

- Are you the woman who is placed in someone's life to remind her of all God has for her?
- Are you the woman who talks friends, sisters, or relatives through one of the most challenging experiences of their lives?
- Are you sound enough in your faith to be the rock that someone else can depend upon?
- Can you be trusted with connecting someone to Christ in the midst of her poor decision making?

Section Application: Live with Ease

Women of God tend to have tenacity and influence in their Christian walks. Through the first two chapters, each sister exhibits a certain level of tenacity and influence.

TENACITY: the state of being persistent in maintaining or seeking something valued or desired; not easily pulled apart.

How does the definition of *tenacity* apply to the women in these two chapters?

_____

_____

_____

INFLUENCE: The act or power of producing an effect, without apparent exertion of force or direct exercise of command.

How does the definition of *influence* apply to the women in these two chapters?

_____

_____

_____

THE WOMEN WITHIN

In each chapter, there is a specific type of woman discussed.
Describe the woman in chapter 1:

_____

_____

_____

Describe the woman in chapter 2:

_____

_____

_____

What characteristics do these women possess that *enhance* their
ability to be used by God?

_____

_____

_____

What characteristics do these women possess that may *hinder* their
ability to be used by God?

_____

_____

_____

What are their greatest flaws? What are their greatest strengths?

_____

_____

_____

If you could give advice to these women, what would it be?

1. Advice for the woman in chapter 1:

_____

_____

_____

_____

_____

2. Advice for the woman in chapter 2:

_____

_____

_____

SCRIPTURAL REFERENCES

Study the following scripture:

"Yea, though I walk through the valley of the shadow of death, I will fear no evil: for thou art with me; thy rod and thy staff they comfort me." (Psalm 23:4 KJV)

What are the key words/terms in this scripture?

_____

_____

_____

How does this scripture apply to the spiritual place that the woman in chapter 1 is in?

_____

_____

_____

Study the following scripture:

"Understand this, my dear brothers and sisters: You must all be quick to listen, slow to speak, and slow to get angry." (James 1:19 NLT)

What are the key words/terms in this scripture?

_____

_____

_____

How does this scripture apply to spiritual place that the woman in chapter 2 is in?

_____

_____

_____

PERSONAL RELEVANCE

Name two ways that you relate to the woman in chapter 1.

1. _____

_____

2. _____

_____

Name two ways that you relate to the woman in chapter 2.

1. _____

_____

2. _____

_____

LOVING YOU THROUGH IT

Now that you have read chapters 1 and 2, reflection is necessary to determine where these women are represented in your life.

Do you have a faithful sister in Christ?   YES   NO

Are you a faithful sister in Christ?   YES   NO

What makes you determine someone's status as a "faithful sister"?

_____

_____

_____

Considering that a faithful sister serves as an accountability partner, what are two things you can do to be a better representation of a sister in Christ?

1. _____

    _____

2. _____

    _____

    _____

How will accomplishing these two goals help your spiritual growth?

_____

_____

_____

Identify and name your faithful sister, and write a note thanking her for being your "ride or die" friend.

* If you do not have a faithful sister, write a note to a friend telling her where you would like to be in Christ and challenging her to hold you accountable.

_____

_____

_____

_____

_____

_____

Building women who are faithful sisters regarding God's Word is a Kingdom goal!

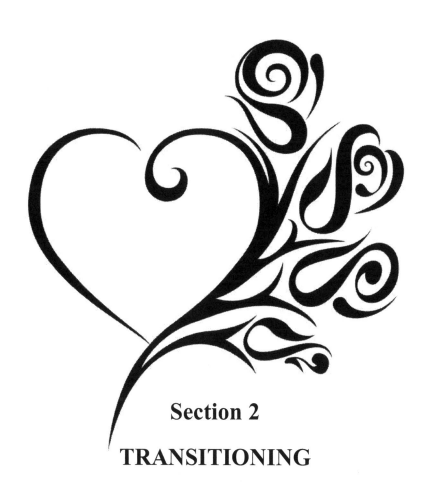

Section 2

TRANSITIONING

THE PURPOSE OF TRANSITIONING

Transition: passage from one state, stage, subject, or place to another.

Have you ever pondered what the necessary steps are to successfully transition? Or thought about the strategy it would take to move smoothly from one place in life to another?

Allowing us to move, God expects us to rise to the occasion and trust His hand while we are in motion. The moments when we're unsure of our purpose, God expects us to seek Him. Transitions challenge us by placing us into predicaments that force us to grow or acknowledge our own personal truths. In warlike fashion, these challenges can leave us surrendering or shouting for victory. They make us examine our hearts and take note of revelations and distractions from our God-given purpose.

In the next few chapters, I acknowledge sisters living through seasons of transition. The in-between stage of life where they experience conflict between who they are and who they are becoming. A time when they are expected to disclose their hearts' deepest secrets while they are still learning them. The time when they must express God's promises while their circumstances remain unmoved. This is a season that consists of many doubts and fears. Sometimes. At other times it consists of belief and trust. It's a double-minded, wishy-washy type of season! Sometimes they believe for others. Sometimes they believe for themselves. But all the time they are learning: about their character flaws, their issues, and the crosses they must bear in life! They have access to this phase for growth, strength, and empowerment.

In this section, three different women will describe aspects and challenges of transitioning. The brokenness. The struggle. The trauma. The growth. The hope. The lessons learned. These sisters determine what it means to deal with transition, what the transition has taught them about themselves, and what they need to address to become who God wants them to be.

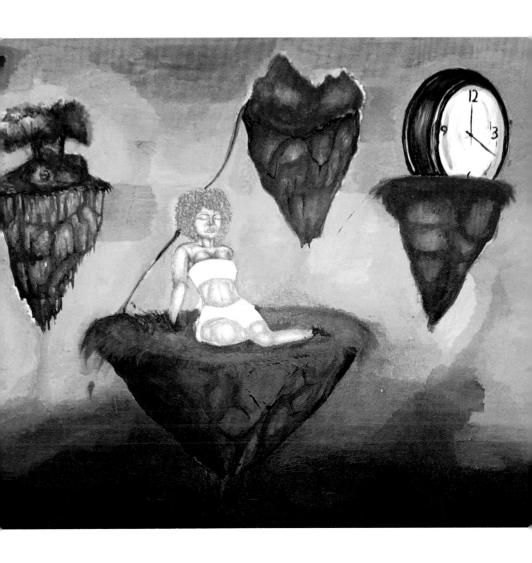

MIND GAMES AND MENTAL SHIFTS

The concept of security plays games with true reality.

Can we ever truly be secure in a position that is dictated by moving pieces?

If my standard is based on the fact that people will transition in and out of this compartment, do I have a reality at all?

The mere thought that this has come to my mind is something that baffles me and makes me question the fate of my life.

Here I am. At this stage in life where everything has become a question mark. And nothing is a definite.

How did I get here?

He left. She's crazy. I want them away. Can't stand to be apart. Need an ear to hear me, but don't want to talk. I have dreams that have been realized, but I yearn for something else.

Where exactly am I in life?

Am I ahead or behind?

Depends on who I compare myself to. But why should I have to make a comparison?

My life seems like a floatation device. Not the large ducks that kids flaunt around their waists and look forward to jumping into the pool with.

My life is more like the floatation devices that sit folded in the hidden compartment of the airplane, awaiting doom.

That feeling when the flight attendant gets on the speaker and says, "In the event of crashing, please take out your floatation device"...I am crashing.

I have crashed.

I tried to escape this reality, but it has caught up with me, and now I am in need of help.

All the help. ANY HELP!

For life has taught me that each level of success comes with a level of pain. But each level of pain makes me feel an inadequacy that I have never experienced before.

A challenge that is unmatched and unmet, until the breakthrough comes.

I await breakthrough.

Tapping into those items that bring me some peace. I try to avoid counter productivity, but sometimes stagnation shreds my soul.

My thought patterns will have me trying anything to silence the whispers of my own heart.

The questions I ask. The WHY? WHEN? HOW?

No whispers given. THEY YELL.

For it is important to channel back to a source that will keep my mentality in a fresh place.

I am in need of fresh water.

For this water I am sitting in has become tainted with the bitterness that I exude when I think of my current state.

The images of others being freed while I still sit. I am salty.

Insulted by the focus that is needed to keep pushing, yet visually I see nothing happening.

I believe it is happening. Somewhere. Just not here. At this moment.

Unsure and conflicted. I stagger; yet I still stand. I'm confused; yet I still believe.

I am striving toward a mark. An unidentified mark. That no natural being can point in the direction of, but I believe it's near.

I know it. I feel it as I crash down, like waves on the shore.

I take the hit for the formation of something beautiful.

I am waiting. I can't wait. I hate waiting.

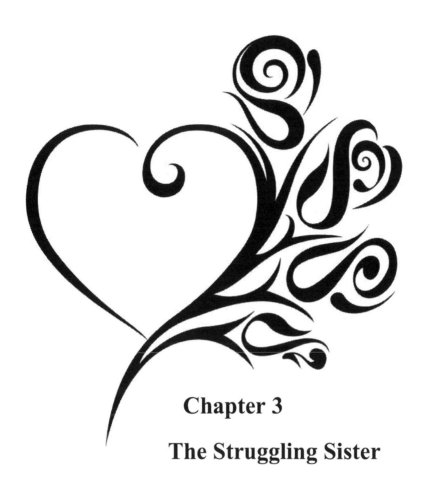

Chapter 3

The Struggling Sister

FLOATING ON BROKEN PIECES

INDECISIVE

I think about my current state of mind and become afraid. I don't believe God is pleased with my indecisiveness, but this in-between phase has me at a standstill. I am searching for myself and God all at the same time. And I don't think I've truly found either one! I constantly question who I am:

- Am I still the version of myself that existed five years ago?
- Am I that young woman who is unsure of herself and becomes whoever people want her to be?
- Or have I grown past that?

I like to think that my relationship with God has gotten closer, but can people see the fruit of it? Can anyone see my growth?

I hope that when people look at me, they can see proof that I've grown closer to God. I hope they can see past my breakdowns and look at my miracles. I feel the direction of my life is changing, but I'm not sure what other people will say. Or, for that matter, what God will say. Lately, He seems distant. It's like I've been reaching for Him but have yet to connect. At times I'm hopeful, but right now life seems bleak. I'm persevering, but this phase is stressful.

Meanwhile, I'm the one who is trying to convince everyone else that their lives will work out. They have no idea I secretly believe my life will not. Am I living a lie? I feel overwhelmed watching other people overcome their trials. Let's face it…forget providing encouragement, right now I need motivation for myself. I need to hear "no weapon formed against you shall prosper," and you have the "power to tread upon serpents, scorpions, and all the power of the enemy." Yet who will speak into my spirit when I have more questions than answers? And when I am full of self-doubt?

I never knew this plan to speak into the lives of others would backfire and leave me lonely. So here I stand, questioning who I am and who I have around me, and feeling silenced all at once.

I prayed. I wept.

I asked God, "Do you hear me?"

I stocked up on sermons. I wept.

I asked God, "Can you see where I am?"

I immersed myself in inspirational music. I wept.

I asked God, "Can you help me?"

I complained. I wept.

And I still felt incomplete.

How is it possible to do this much work and still feel no shift? I was working so hard at trying to hear the voice of God that I forgot about it existing in many other forms. His voice did not only exist as a faint tone of stillness, but it could possibly be the firm, subtle voice of my sister. That raspy, melodic whisper that shook me when I cried out, "I don't know what I'm doing!" God began to use her to speak plainly about my life. She was able to speak to my lack of peace and my mistrust of people. She was sent to check my spirit. When I needed her, God allowed her to be present.

Spiritual Application of Purpose #5

Acknowledge When God Uses Other Forms of Speaking

- God can provide guidance and direction using multiple forms of media.

- When you seek Him, take note of how He speaks to you. Does He use the voices of others, sermons, dreams, visions, or songs? Does He allow you to give others the advice you need?
- How God speaks to you is individually packaged for your benefit.

NOTHING LEFT TO GIVE

I was too proud to let the world see my weaknesses but too damaged to not show it to my sister. Afraid, I doubted God's ability to turn my situation around. "Maybe I will not get to greater," I thought to myself. The picture of a new relationship, an amazing job, healing from my brokenness, and a fresh start was not surfacing, and I felt like the mental attacks were growing stronger each day. I was getting weak. I had no strength to "fight the good fight," and I felt like I was losing. Losing my mind, my dignity, and my breath. I was suffocating.

And then I told God, "I have nothing left to give." I meant it. I wanted Him to see my sorrowful, burdened heart and relieve me of this worry. I wanted to believe again. I wanted to trust that all things were working for me. I wanted to not bear the weight of my burdens. I wanted to let all of it go to God. So I did. I let it go, and in that moment I felt God take over. Figuratively speaking, it felt like a cold breeze on a hot summer's day. No, seriously. My soul, which was dry and bothered, became refreshed. No longer burdened with living a lie, I was free to admit I was not okay. This was the first time I acknowledged outwardly that I needed help.

"That's why I take pleasure in my weaknesses, and in the insults, hardships, persecutions, and troubles that I suffer for Christ. For when I am weak, then I am strong." (2 Corinthians 12:10 NLT)

I believed that God was taking on my burdens. He began to help me get the mess that I was making back together. When I admitted I needed God, He helped me to get friendships, intentions, and standards back on the right track!

PUSH: FOR HER AND FOR YOU

I believe God allowed me to go through my negative circumstances for the sake of testimony. But I acknowledge no one thinks of that while they are going through the circumstances! God wants us to live the lessons...behind closed doors and in front of other people. Bearing burdens can be useful for someone else.

While going through this trial, I wanted to disappear. I could not fathom God using any of this to bless anyone, but that's EXACTLY what God wanted to do! He wanted to me to tell the truth about my situation and to be transparent about it all. God wanted me to speak out about the struggle and the distractions and admit to being hypocritical. To get closer to being healed, I had to discuss the tests I failed and speak intently about the ones I passed.

Spiritual Application of Purpose #6

Speak the Truth, Even When It Hurts to Say It
- It may seem easier to hide your thoughts when you are questioning your life, but it will make you feel isolated.
- Expose yourself. Do not be afraid to be who you are...flaws and all!
- Your loved ones, who are living according to God's purpose, will already know you are struggling and will have been praying for your breakthrough. Find out which loved ones are praying for you, ask God what you can reveal to them and let them hold you accountable for what you can share!

SURRENDERING IT ALL

God was trying to walk me into freedom. No longer a hostage, He was asking me to do two things: trust someone with my emotions and encourage someone else through their own emotions. God was forcing me to become accountable for the thoughts I was having and requiring me to express them. Actions and thoughts.

God wanted me to acknowledge my daily struggle: be comfortable or surrender? Exposing myself to my sister would make her the vessel used to refresh my mind and give me hope. I needed to trust her, allow her to hold my innermost thoughts, and let her redirect me to God.

Where I lacked faith, she would provide me with clarity.

Where I lacked drive, she would give me momentum.

I needed to acknowledge my sister, she needed to acknowledge me, and we needed to acknowledge God. For He had, and has always had, everything under control. The good, the bad, and the ugly. It would all work out for my good.

"And we know that all things work together for good to them that love God, to them who are called according to his purpose." (Romans 8:28 KJV)

This trial would push me to help others, while I learned to allow my sister to help me. She would help me to believe while I struggled waiting for signs. I'm thankful for the listening ear of my sister, but I hope this season's expiration date is coming soon!

"Saying, Father, if thou be willing, remove this cup from me: nevertheless not my will, but thine, be done." (Luke 22:42 KJV)

MAY YOU "LOVE THROUGH" THESE QUESTIONS:

COULD YOU BE HER? The Struggling Sister

- Are you the woman actively trying to find God?
- Do you often question who you are, but hide your questions about yourself from loved ones?
- Are you willing to admit the areas you need help in? And can you expose those areas to a loved one in order to release that burden from your life?

LAQUESHA'S REFLECTION

STILL LEARNING

People say my type is rare

Very firm but fair

Slightly confused but yet still there

I pretend I know all my strengths and scares

However, my dreams give me sense that I'm stronger than I'm aware

So my friendships and God

Intertwine messages that I should be hearing through my ears

So someday the woman that I'm supposed to be I will see in the mirror

Still learning

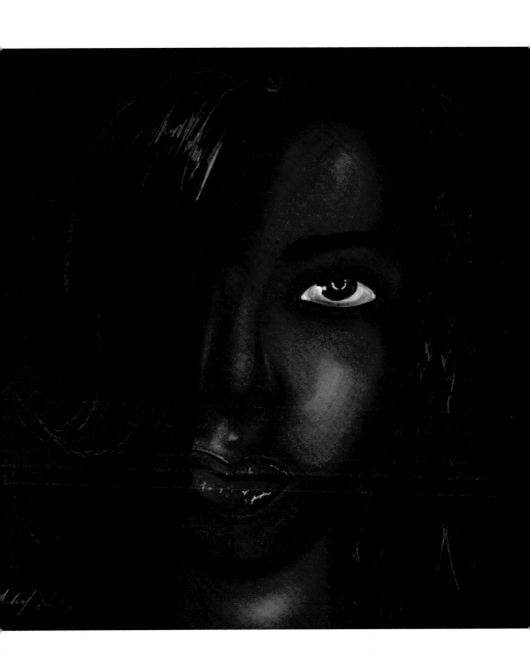

SUCCESSFUL INTRUDER

You broke into this heart of mine and ran rampant through its halls

Roughshod throughout each room, breaking down walls

Tearing into the drywall I put up years ago

To protect and isolate the structures of my spirit

No alarm set off. I wasn't aware of the assailant that unarmed my being,

Nor the damage you would be capable of doing

You made an entrance. Later you would make a hellish exit,

Inspecting my worth and estimating how much damage I had suffered

You guessimated my life's meaning

In your eyes, I serve a tangible purpose

You direct, and I fall in line.

Orders upon orders to get me aesthetically pleasing; yet I never seemed satisfied

Some would call my hungry soul a pit

Money pit. Attention pit. Love pit. You name it, I sought after it. Until the day came when my input grew greater than you could afford.

That was the day your thieving fate became reality and you stole from me

Walked boldly into my space and demanded what you felt entitled to.

You couldn't help yourself

And I…I allowed you into that space.

Not paying attention to the sketches you made or the notes you took

When I talked, you listened intently.

When I walked, you followed.

Admiring my movement while planning moves on your own.

You were slick.

Put in the code to my heart, walked into my life, and chiseled away at the meanings of this season

I'm bewildered. Lost at the audacity, and shocked that it was you.

I would've never guessed it would be you

Depleting my value and forcing me to renovate

I'm now upgrading my life because of you

The cost is high, but the payoff will be endless

It's necessary

Now that you've run away with my outdated fixings

This market doesn't have use for what you stole, other than stories of what was

Sadness sinks in as I realize that I will have to start again

But joy overtakes me as I consider the endless possibilities of a new beginning

Your larceny has created opportunity

For this I say thank you.

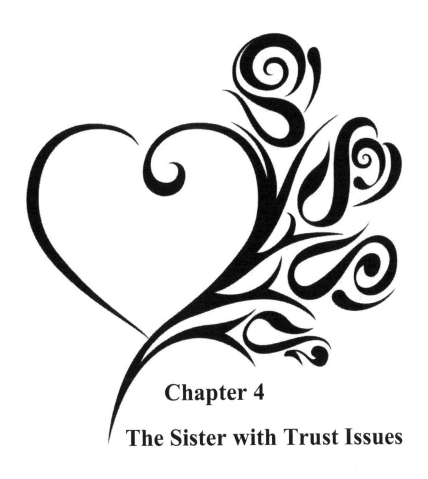

Chapter 4

The Sister with Trust Issues

HIDDEN BETRAYAL

LOST IN THE PAST

Have you ever felt blindsided? Like someone bamboozled your senses and attacked at the most inopportune time? My life has landed me here, trusting no one and trying to shake bitterness. Inside this wall of emotions, I have decided that I am safer here. Without the need to step outside of my comfort zone, I have created a space that is comfortable for me. Yet I recognize it imprisons me with the stagnation. I feel trapped. One hand balled into a fist, and the other hand waving in the air for help. I'm not sure what I want.

Miserable, yet trying to please everyone.

Confused, yet acting like I have everything under control.

I'm in a state of purgatory. Not out in the light, but not quite in darkness. I have succumbed to the state of life that no one wants to live in…I'm stuck in the middle. I am lukewarm.

"I know thy works, that thou art neither cold nor hot: I would thou wert cold or hot. So then because thou art lukewarm, and neither cold nor hot, I will spue thee out of my mouth." (Revelation 3:15–16 KJV)

I know that I should not be stuck and that I am called to be so much more, but I have to be honest when I speak about the fear of stepping into more.

What does "more" look like?

How does "more" benefit me?

And why has God made "more" seem so stressful?

I often think about the ones who told me that I could be something greater, do something amazing, and I think, "Where did they go?" Where are those individuals who vowed to be with me through the trials of my life? Where were they when my heart was broken, or my spirit was being crushed? My heart still sinks when I think of the hurt I have endured, and then it dawns on me…I haven't seen them since! And I'm not over it!

I'm not over the abandonment. We were always together, always discussing the future and continually talking about God's ways…then they left. Mumbling something about confronting their "demons," I guess they decided demon chasing was better without me. But now I'm stuck. Trying to figure out what "confronting your demons" means, I am faced with the harsh reality that I don't know what I need to confront!

This should be easy, but I do not know where to begin! Truth is, doing this task was easier with someone else. They told me what was wrong with me, and I worked hard to see it. Now I am expected to do this by myself? The reality is, my relationship was crippling. Taking all of my spiritual attention, it taught me how to be selfish, inconsiderate, and broken. I needed a refreshing word and healing…spiritual healing.

Have you ever been there?

In a place where you realize that the person you counted on to help you grow only helped you to manifest all the negative attributes about yourself?

There I was asking myself, "What are my good traits?" I was in a space where I had to admit I had very little positivity to give to anyone. All I could see was my brokenness. Completely alarmed at this thought, I asked God, "What do You see in me?" I knew that I was taking a chance, but I needed to know! A hard pill to swallow when you are told, "You've been so busy analyzing other people that you failed to analyze who you are." Man. So here I am. Jotting down the struggles that I have had in life…the childhood hurt, the generational curses, the pain from relationships, and the emotional scarring. I was beginning to uncover the hidden places that have kept my heart captive. Maybe addressing them would help? Is this "confronting your demons"?

LET IT OUT

I need God to show me a way out of this frame of mind. I am not sure how I got here, but somewhere down the line, my demons and my skeletons took hold of my progress in life. Yes, I said demons and skeletons. Demons because some of my experiences have lent themselves to being conducive to demonic activity. I admit to being in the wrong places and hanging with people who had the wrong spirits, and those decisions put me in a place where I became vulnerable to demonic attack.

I didn't know.

I did not know that each time I failed a test of temptation, I became weaker to Satan's attack. My will for God's way was growing weaker. I did not know that each time I performed the opposite of God's standard, I was actively working on behalf of Satan and minimizing my Christ-like character.

"Anyone who isn't with me opposes me, and anyone who isn't working with me is actually working against me." (Luke 11:23 NLT)

And then comes the skeletons, the past experiences that I have allowed to pile up in the background of my life, crowding my personal space. Full of mistakes and embarrassments, I realize that instead of burying them, I have memorialized moments. I have celebrated the moments that I should have released from my memory and now see the hinderance to my life. I need God to help me with the strategy to fight these demonic attacks and get rid of the skeletons in my life.

Spiritual Application of Purpose #7:

Ask God for a Strategy

- Victory requires God's strategy, so it would behoove you to ask Him for it!
- Be specific in your prayers when asking for strategy. Ask God what you should look for and how He expects you to respond.
- Do not assume that asking for strategy will give you a quick and automatic win! Some battles are won quickly, and others can span a lifetime. The goal is to get to a place where you can trust God's lead and follow His word of direction.

Some may think it's taboo to acknowledge Satan's ability to attack, but I have to acknowledge his tactics to fight effectively. Just like armies studying previous attacks, I have to take note of what Satan does, how he does it, and what response I need to have to be victorious. I need to paint an authentic picture of who I should be versus who I am during spiritual attack. This is serious! I need to expose my personal temptations and ask God to show me how the enemy sways me away from the will of God.

In my case, the temptation has always been the opposite sex. The stumbling block that I seem ignorant to every time! Hindering my progress, I have allowed them to lead me to places I should not have been, talk me out of my dreams, walk me away from blessings, and take me into a place of spiritual darkness. It shakes me as I say this, but I have failed this test over and over again. Struggling with my own self-worth, I have let men speak things into my spirit that no woman should accept. I have received their love while they were in other intimate relationships. I have settled for second and third place, and at times, no place at all. I have cried tears of frustration when I thought of all my heart had given when it didn't work out. In spite of the fact that I knew it wasn't going to work, I gave of myself. I gave in to this area of attack, and now I am paying for it.

The enemy knows that I would rather hide these events in my heart. I would rather not speak of the captivity that my heart and mind are in. The hurt that I have tried to hide and the stumbling blocks that I have allowed Satan to use frequently…today, they stop! Today I am declaring an end to them! I am letting myself out of this trap, and I will begin to live freely. Recognizing my main attack, I will succeed at the next test! Challenges are exactly that…challenges. They were not created to rule me, I was meant to dominate them. Today, I will. I will no longer fear the unknown; greatness cannot come from convenience! I need to step out and push through my discomfort! These attacks are coming because of who I am in God and what I am destined to become.

"But anyone who obeys God's laws and teaches them will be called great in the Kingdom of Heaven." (Matthew 5:19b NLT)

FIGHT TO BREAK FREE

I used to be nervous to speak about my mistakes. The fact that I'm speaking of them now is a breakthrough! I believed that everyone's lives were so much more structured than mine. You could not tell me that other people were experiencing the same struggles I was. Their lives looked sound. They had sound jobs, sound relationships, sound families, sound children, and sound Christian spirits. Mine was everything but sound.

In fact, my life seemed more like a roller coaster than a straight paved street. But who wants to admit to that? Who wants to admit that, due to failures, the fantasy of who I would be by this age is in stark contrast with reality? I created an expectation for my life that pushed me into a corner. I was taking punches. I wonder if other people see this? Can they see the misery that I am really living? Or are they buying the images I portray?

Convincing myself and others has become the game I'm playing, but I'm tired. I secretly hope someone sees through it and goes to God for a miracle. I need it. I need God to get me out of this state. I know He can do it, I just struggled with asking. I needed God to deliver me. I needed God to heal me. I needed God to help me release grudges and offenses. So, in tears, I asked. I asked Him to help me apologize and rectify situations that I helped to deteriorate. And I asked Him to work on my heart. I wanted a miracle, and I was willing to risk it all to move forward from this space.

Have you ever been there?

Where you wanted God to move so badly that you were willing to do anything for Him to change your situation?

There I was, asking God to help me so I could be who He intended me to be. I was willing to move forward. I wanted God to present me with the opportunity. This time, I was ready. I can't wait to see what He does!

MAY YOU "LOVE THROUGH" THESE QUESTIONS:

COULD YOU BE HER? The Sister with Trust Issues

- Are you the woman whose destiny is driven by those who are around you? Can you identify people who may be your downfall?
- Are you able to identify areas of your life where the enemy wins often? Can you surrender those areas to God?
- Are you in a place where you desire to win in those areas more than you desire hiding those areas?

CRYSTAL'S REFLECTION

Our rearview mirror is an important feature, standard in vehicles. It helps you see what's behind you, to gauge how you move forward.

This, however, can be tricky. You need it to be appropriately positioned. And you mustn't stay glued to it, though you should check it often, or there will be problems ahead of you.

This is our life! We have "rearviews" of our past.

In order to continue to walk as new creations, we should reflect on past events to be sure we are going in the right direction.

But as with the rearview mirrors, if we stay stuck looking at our past (the who we were, why he left, or the things we thought were so great that we no longer have), we will not be able to navigate, let alone thrive, in our future.

JODANA'S REFLECTION

"And you will seek Me and find Me, when you search for Me with all your heart." (Jeremiah 29:13 NKJV)

"'The LORD is my portion,' says my soul, 'Therefore I hope in Him!' The LORD is good to those who wait for Him, To the soul who seeks Him." (Lamentations 3:24–25 NKJV)

Remember, the TRUE FULFILLMENT IS GOD, THROUGH HIS SON JESUS CHRIST, and only that! Continue (or go back to) seeking God only. And not what He can do for you in material, tangible, and vain things. Continue to trust and rest in God. Continue to seek Him with all your heart and soul. Continue loving God for who He is and how much He loves you, and remembering Him for saving us! Love on God! Trust in God! Because He is loving you through and teaching you through! When you do this, you will have true fulfillment in Him. You will find true love for yourself. You will have true love for yourself. Because of your seeking and love in God. And in God alone.

Remember, seek and desire God more than anything!

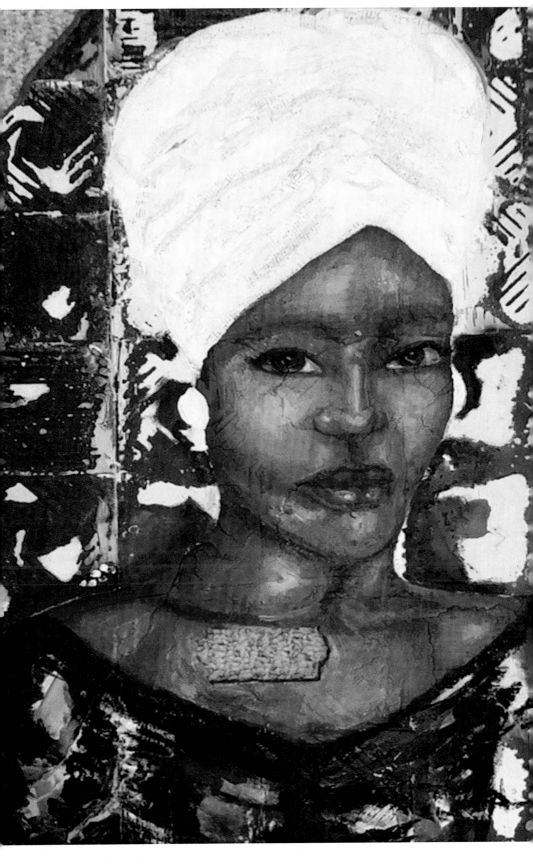

VISION UNSEEN

On the outside looking in.

I've been there and can see your future from this space.

You don't see past where you are now, but let me give you a glimpse

It's beautiful at this location.

Afar off, but its beauty outweighs the path taken to get there.

You will remember it all, but you'll have to be conscious of the promises that God filled on the way.

I've been there. In the awkward stage of life. Not quite transitioned out of misery, but not fully seeing victory.

You keep walking toward God's marvelous light.

There is safety in His presence, and you have found His sweet spot.

Take advantage of the instructions given, they will help you navigate the waters in which God intends to pull out of you His will.

I see past your potential into a faithful arena, where God can shift your atmosphere.

Molding you into who He created you to be.

It hurts, but it'll be worth it.

I am a testament to the works that God can do.

One move at a time, He elevates your thinking and reveals your true spirit.

His spirit and who He really is.

'Tis so sweet to trust in Jesus.

He is loving and loves you enough to send someone to you that knows the way.

He is the way. But how am I supposed to know how crucial that statement is without an indication that God is not to be played with.

Such a colorful spirit.

You exude purple, white, and red. The colors of royalty, purity, and the blood.

May He cover this season, as He once covered me

May He give me words of wisdom to expound to you, that you may be able to learn through listening and not merely doing

I've been there.

A penetrating place where I felt strangled by circumstances and wandered aimlessly at times

I heard God's unfamiliar voice and ran wild with my own devices

Don't be like me. Listen. Follow. Obey. Willingly.

I've been there. Holding the heavy hand that life has dealt you.

Know that you do not have to travel this alone. I am here.

To be the attentive ear that I had. The sight that I wish I could see. And the voice of reason that seemingly makes no sense at all.

You trust me because I've been there, and I trust God.

To lead you to your destination. To give me wisdom for your journey.

Acknowledging that your life's strife is for the cause of Christ, so you need not be distracted

Stay focused and make it through this stint

With tunnel vision on pleasing God.

He'll always be there.

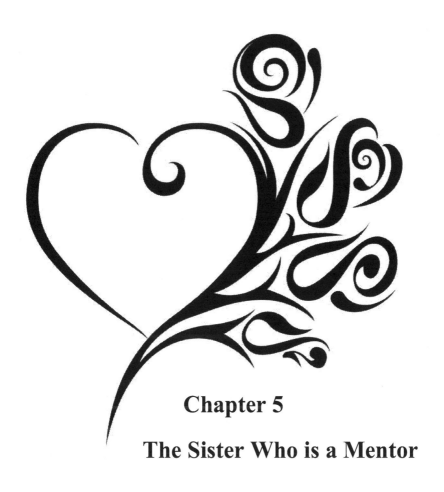

Chapter 5

The Sister Who is a Mentor

TUNNELED SUPPORT

FIRSTHAND EXPERIENCE

"I lit up the room. It occurred so quickly. I felt like I couldn't control it." That's how I began my conversation with this young lady. She was so hurt, and I immediately recognized where she was. I'd been in that place before…lost and hurt. Such a definitive moment, when it seems like the life that you have built is crumbling in front of you. Everything she thought she stood for, she is now reconsidering. "I never will" has become "I can't believe I'm considering this." I have been there.

I sat listening to this young lady tell her story as she cried tears of sorrow. She kept referring to herself, but I knew inside this was also my story. I thought, "She will be amazed at the similarities and the traits that make us kindred spirits." I am her. The child whose childhood produced bitterness. The lost young lady hiding behind the badge of independence. And the hurt woman who questions her identity. I've been her. I have been in the very place of loneliness that she is in, asking the very same questions she ponders, and wishing someone would help me. They did.

I guess now it is my turn.

It's my turn to share my testimony and reveal the phases of life that God has blessed me to get through. Reminiscing brings tears to my eyes, and I am drawn back to that place. I empathize with her. The feeling of longing to be accepted while being completely confused. I have been there. I have struggled with my share of the blues: my weight, my health, my family relationships, my history with men, my insecurities, and my lack of understanding. I knew all too well what it meant to be in bondage. So I instantly recognized it on her. She was overtaken by her thoughts, and they made her wonder if she would ever get beyond this day. She would. She would one day become a pillar to another young woman and give her the same advice I am going to give...but today is my day. My day to tell her that she will be all right. And I knew that because I am.

"But Jesus said, 'No, go home to your family, and tell them everything the Lord has done for you and how merciful he has been.'" (Mark 5:19 NLT)

EMPATHY AND FAITH

I cannot pinpoint the day that I realized life circumstances were temporary, but on what seemed to be the worst day of my life, I laid on my floor crying and contemplating life. The minutes turned into hours, and before I knew it, I had very little voice left to cry, and I was thinking my life had been useless!

Have you ever been there?

In a place where you struggle to find one effective area in your life?

There I was trying to find it, and none of the options were working. Maybe my job is great...but it could always be better. Maybe my friendships are amazing...but they could always be more transparent. Maybe my spiritual life was increasing...but I could always be more consistent. I was struggling in every area. Honestly, the more I tried to make things work my way, the more they fell apart. God had to be laughing at my attempts to find solutions, because I was running out of ideas. *There has to be another way*, I thought. *I just don't know what it is!* I felt hopeless and heartbroken.

Spiritual Application of Purpose #8:

Let Your Heart Break

- Everyone will give you advice on how to keep yourself together, but who gives you information on how to properly let your heart grieve?
- Tell yourself, "When I am wounded, it is appropriate to be brokenhearted."
- In the moments that you have admitted to heartbreak, know that you need healing. Admit to being brokenhearted, but don't stay there!

"He heals the brokenhearted and bandages their wounds" (Psalm 147:3 NLT)

With little-known options, I was desperate and spoke out. This woman asked me, "How are you doing?" And I broke down crying. I was so glad someone finally asked me, because the burden I was carrying was more than I knew what to do with. So I told her everything! I wasn't sure if it was more than she bargained for or if she was strategic in the question she asked, but I didn't care...I needed to let it out.

That day, I poured my heart out to the godly woman who sat patiently and listened intently. I cried out, story after story, and she nodded. All she did was reach in her purse for a tissue, but I felt her heart. She knew I needed this release, and she was here for it. When I was completely deflated, a stranger saw through to my soul and said, "I understand." Then she shared her story of pain and anguish, the trials that led her to know Jesus, and the following words, "One day you will be required to uplift another woman as I have uplifted you. For this burden was given to you as a gift to share with others."

Spiritual Application of Purpose #9:

Be an Intentional Listener—You May Have to Share Your Testimony

- Being a good listener is a burden to bear. It calls for you to listen with your heart and spirit, rather than just your ears. What is their heart expressing?
- If you let them vent, you have made an internal vow to pray over what they speak, uplift their spirit, and push them to grow. You are now responsible for their level of accountability.
- Know that not all listening sessions will be a moment for you to speak, but you should be mindful that your time to share your testimony will come. Be ready!

It seems backward the way God uses tribulations to bring us closer to Him, but His ways are strategic. I would have never imagined that the most gut-wrenching moments of my life would be the moments that would give me insight into the mind of God. In those hours, while the tears filled my eyes, I sought God the most. I believe He had to get me to a place where I had no one else to lean on but Him. It was then that I learned to trust Him. I never knew what that meant before. God was teaching me, and I am grateful for those lessons. And now as I stand in front of this young lady, she reminds me of the very conversation I had with my stranger many years ago. Here I am. Offering this woman wisdom. Just as the lady predicted. Who knew this day would come?

TOUGH LOVE

In between her cries, I reminded her of purpose. "Do you know God has a plan for all of this?" I whispered to her. She did not see it, but she is destined for greatness. God does not allow people to go through challenging situations without purpose. If I can just get her to see the blessings in this storm, she would soon realize the privilege she has been granted. She was chosen for this moment. Like Job's life was presented to Satan to test, her life was being presented as well. Now what would she do with it?

Challenging her was God's challenge to me. It was tough to revisit my past, but He was calling me to assist someone with her present. I had to examine if I was really healed.

- Did I take the time to sit in my experience?
- Have I released all the hurt and pain to God?
- Have I admitted to all parts of the story?
- Was I able to own my role and how it contributed to my growth or lack of it?

God was asking me to be transparent while this young woman shared each gut-wrenching detail of her story. I reflected on my life. I remembered the faces. I felt the emotions. And I began to smile at the thought that God got me through it. With that, I had faith that He would get her through this as well. She just needed the faith.

Spiritual Application of Purpose #10:

Reflect on God's Victories in Your Life

- What has God brought you through that can be used as a testimony?
- When analyzing victories, what did God reveal about YOU? What characteristics did the battle get rid of that were hindering your personal or spiritual growth?
- It is easy to point out the flaws and growth areas of others, but God wants us to focus on our own!

I told her that today would be a monumental day for her. She needed to mark this on a calendar! Although today seems gruesome, I wanted her to imagine herself free of the pain and well into her new season. This day is the beginning of something great. God decided that she was ready to be launched into her purpose. And sometimes launching is painful.

Explaining the process of launching a rocket into space, I talked about the stages it goes through to prepare. Each engine has its purpose, from thrusting to separation to engagement, each engine goes through a phase that allows it to continue on its trajectory. I asked her, "If something as materialistic as a rocket has phases of launching, why do you think you won't need phases to become who God has created you to be?" She looked bewildered.

LEAD ME BACK

I guess I'm unofficially an mentor now. This holds a lot of weight, and I had to uphold a standard. I couldn't choose to straddle the fence anymore. I had to pick a side. God's way or Satan's way?

"But you, Timothy, are a man of God; so run from all these evil things. Pursue righteousness and a godly life, along with faith, love, perseverance, and gentleness. Fight the good fight for the true faith. Hold tightly to the eternal life to which God has called you, which you have declared so well before many witnesses." (1 Timothy 6:11–12 NLT)

Funny how things work out, because I felt like I needed advice as much as she did. I still had lessons to learn and circumstances to travel through, but that did not exempt me from God's need to tell my story. He had brought me out of my trial for a reason, and I had to be courageous and boldly proclaim that she would make it out victoriously too. Just as God provided for me, He would provide for her! For the very essence of the breakthrough she was waiting on begins with this painful situation. Later, I texted her the following message:

"He does hear your heart's cry! Love you, and I am so proud of the woman you have become through this process and the courage you have demonstrated while going through it... Know that our Father in heaven is well pleased. Be still and know that He is God and Mighty in the Midst of Thee!!"

MAY YOU "LOVE THROUGH" THESE QUESTIONS:

COULD YOU BE HER? The Sister Who Is a Mentor

- Are you the woman who God uses as an example of overcoming?
- Have you been around women who are living through situations that you have come out of victoriously?
- Are you willing to encourage them to see the bright side of their troublesome situation, while holding them accountable to God? Even if it means you expose your own flawed life?

SUMMER'S REFLECTION

Listening with a spirit of discernment and not anticipation.
A word given from Lord God above.

Very clear instructions, but easier said than done.

A journey called "LIFE" traveled with ups, downs, and everything in between.

But God.

As I reflect on my past, present, and future, I am more aware of the need for Godly Community.

Pastor Michael Todd said it best when he spoke about creating an inner circle of people closest to you, where you can live to fulfill God's purpose.

While there have been many times I wanted to shout and scream out of despair, I have been fortunate to have the right sisters, at just the right place, at the right time.

As I continue to press toward the mark of excellence or living in my truth, I believe firmly God is speaking through my sister with this book.

To discern the next sister's struggle is to operate in love and communicate life lessons only a sister can give.

"Always sisters, always friends."

"Be careful for nothing: but in every thing by prayer and supplication with thanksgiving let your requests be made known unto God." (Philippians 4:6 KJV)

Section Application: Transitioning

Women of God tend to persevere through struggles that can help them to grow. Through chapters 3 and 4, each sister reveals a level of struggle and perseverance.

PERSEVERANCE: continued effort to do or achieve something despite difficulties, failure, or opposition; the act of persevering.

How does the definition of *perseverance* apply to the women in chapters 3, 4, and 5?

_____

_____

_____

How can you apply the definition of *perseverance* to your own life?

_____

_____

_____

THE WOMAN WITHIN

In each chapter there is a specific type of woman discussed. Describe the woman in chapter 3:

_____

_____

_____

Describe the woman in chapter 4:

_____

_____

_____

Describe the woman in chapter 5:

_____

_____

_____

What characteristics do these women possess that *enhance* their ability to be used by God?

_____

_____

_____

What characteristics do these women possess that may *hinder* their ability to be used by God?

_____

_____

_____

What are their greatest flaws? What are their greatest strengths?

_____

_____

_____

If you could give advice to these women, what would it be?

    1.   Advice for the woman in chapter 3:

_____

_____

    2.   Advice for the woman in chapter 4:

_____

_____

    3.   Advice for the woman in chapter 5:

_____

_____

_____

SCRIPTURAL REFERENCES

Study the following scripture:

"That's why I take pleasure in my weaknesses, and in the insults, hardships, persecutions, and troubles that I suffer for Christ. For when I am weak, then I am strong." (2 Corinthians 12:10 NLT)

What are the key words/terms in this scripture?

_____

_____

_____

How does this scripture apply to the spiritual place that the woman in chapter 3 is in?

_____

_____

_____

Study the following scripture:

"Anyone who isn't with me opposes me, and anyone who isn't working with me is actually working against me." (Luke 11:23 NLT)

What are the key words/terms in this scripture?

_____

_____

_____

How does this scripture apply to the spiritual place that the woman in chapter 4 is in?

_____

_____

_____

Study the following scripture:

"He heals the brokenhearted and bandages their wounds." (Psalm 147:3 NLT)

What are the key words/terms in this scripture?

_____

_____

_____

How does this scripture apply to the spiritual place that the woman in chapter 5 is in?

_____

_____

_____

PERSONAL RELEVANCE

Name four ways that you relate to the women in chapters 3, 4, and 5.

1. _____

_____

2. _____

_____

3. _____

_____

4. _____

_____

LOVING YOU THROUGH IT

Now that you've read these three chapters, reflection is necessary.

Discuss a time when you questioned yourself or your purpose in life. During that time, did you have a woman in your life who lifted you?

_____

_____

_____

Learning to trust can be difficult. Identify a woman you trust and describe why you trust her.

_____

_____

_____

What events in your life have made it hard for you to trust?

_____

_____

_____

How do those events hinder your ability to trust God?

_____

_____

_____

When you are living for God, a testimony should come from every storm of life. Write a testimony that could help other women overcome.

_____

_____

_____

Will you be able to share this testimony with other women? YES or NO

Growth is continuous. Write a spiritual goal you thought of while reading the last three chapters.

_____

_____

_____

Much like the experience of the woman in chapter 5, name three women you know that have mastered the goal you have identified.

1. _____

_____

2. _____

_____

3. _____

_____

Write down four questions you can ask them about the goal you are trying to accomplish.

1. _____

_____

2. _____

_____

_____

3. _____

   _____

   _____

4. _____

   _____

   _____

Interview those three women and ask them about their experience in this area.

AFTER INTERVIEWING: What do you now know, about this goal, that you didn't think of prior to interviewing those who have experienced
this?_____

_____

_____

_____

_____

_____

_____

Transitioning women from novice to experienced is a Kingdom goal!

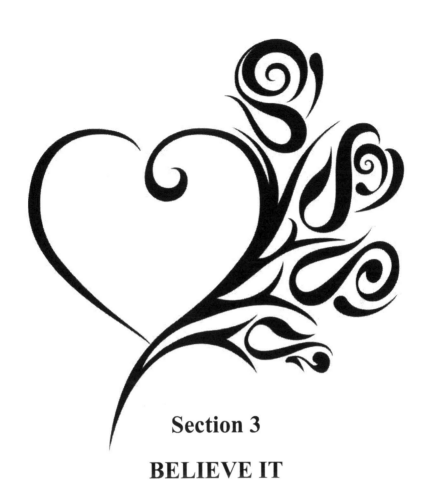

Section 3

BELIEVE IT

THE PURPOSE OF BELIEVING

BELIEF: something that is accepted, considered to be true, or held as an opinion; something believed.

What's in your belief system? And do you believe God when He says you can have your heart's desire?

In the next few chapters, you will examine sisters who are commanded by God to be messengers to other sisters. They are challenged to put their words into action and help others believe in the God who delivers. Assisting other sisters can help to refocus their own lives and enable them to become living examples of God's power working within them.

"Now unto him that is able to do exceeding abundantly above all that we ask or think, according to the power that worketh in us..." *(Ephesians 3:20 KJV)*

These women are being led to guide other women through their process by sharing the lessons they have learned firsthand! They are living examples of how God leads us to sisters who have been in similar situations and gives them the wisdom and knowledge to help others succeed.

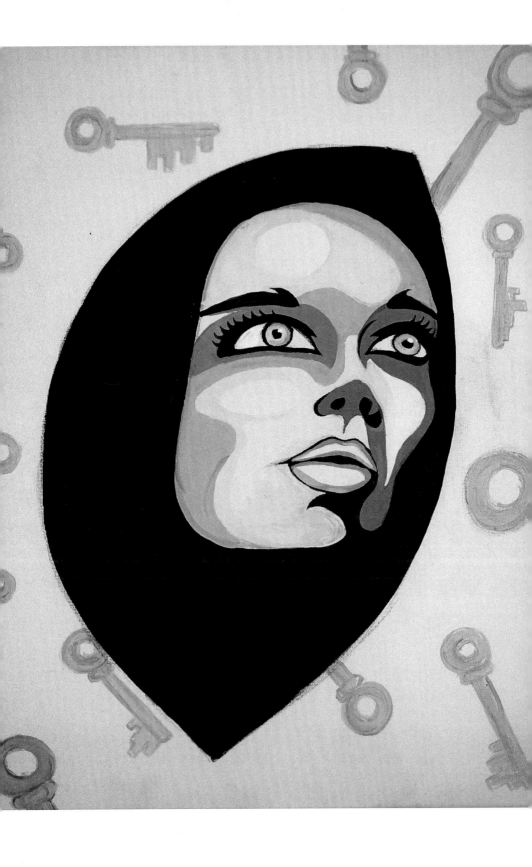

TRUTH'S BRIDGE

Blindfolded, you walk across the bridge entitled "Your New Life"

Scared to death. At least a fleshly death.

This walk will require a different type of faith. A leap that transcends anything you have ever heard God give you.

He expects you to do WHAT?!

How could He possibly anticipate that you would be equipped to handle the brevity of this next assignment?

Your breathing is shorter and deeper than you can ever imagine

Like the height of this mountain has shocked your system into believing you are at high altitude

Yet, spiritually, you are

A place where stairclimbing is a norm and finding yourself breathless is an expectation

You await chaos and find that peace follows you

Second to the line leader, when He stops, you stop

Whether you want to or not, for He promised to get you to your destination, and you are still not there

Whining while walking

Watching and praying

You trust Him, but are nosy enough to ask multiple questions

Praise God it doesn't hinder the process!

The questions about the walk, the way, the direction, the timing, the resources.

Praise God it hasn't hindered the process!

For every answer I am given resides in the realm of truth

An honesty and openness that assures me until the next season

The next move

The next question. Why did you do this, God? How did you know I needed this, God? What do you expect me to do, God? Where are you taking me, God? When will all you've shown me be fulfilled, God?

Full of wonders and favor. I thank you, God, for this moment.

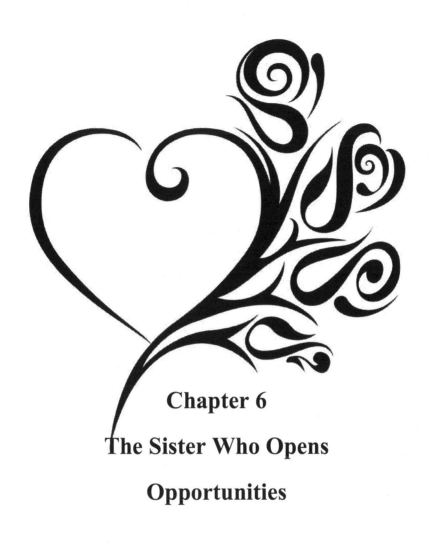

Chapter 6

The Sister Who Opens

Opportunities

OPEN DOORS

ON THE LOOKOUT

I'm excited! I am seeing God move in a unique way in my life. Everything He said to me is coming true. The dreams I had, the visions I saw, the blessings I prayed for...they are all coming to fruition. I could say I saw this coming, but a part of me still had doubts. I'm not sure why, but I questioned God. I wanted to know if He would actually come through for me, asking if He had more for me than this? Each time I asked, He revealed pieces of what was to come.

He gave me warnings.

He gave me directions.

And He gave me insight.

They were all needed, because I had no idea what was happening. I needed to know what God expected me to do. I needed to know if He thought my responses were appropriate. Now I'm starting to see that my labor was not in vain...God was telling me to trust Him, and now, I am starting to see why!

Have you ever been there?

When you are beginning to see the promises of God manifested in your life?

There I was tearing up at the thought that my season of sowing is over and my season of reaping has begun! I have waited so long to see the promises He told me: the blessings, the open doors, the resources, the peace, and the joy. And now I finally see it!

USHER ME THROUGH

I've always been the woman who carried burdens for others. *If you need money, call me. If you need advice, call me. And if you need to vent, call me.* This had been happening for many years until the season came when I needed someone to support me. That's when I felt the most alone. How is it possible to be so many things to so many people and not have someone there for me? I was bewildered. Crying at night, I begged God to send someone who could be my shoulder to cry on. That's when God granted me a new sister. She came into my life at precisely the right time! Exuding strength and wisdom, she began to uplift me. She gifted me with a listening ear and became an accountability partner.

Spiritual Application of Purpose #11:

Find an Accountability Partner

- As you mature in Christ, you will need someone who will challenge you to stay consistent with biblical standards.
- Be prepared for your accountability partner to disagree when you are doing something outside the will of God. True accountability partners will check you...in love.

God was bringing me into a place of maturity that required a sister who matched that level. I felt like we were one in the same: both trying to get closer to God and wanting our lives to exemplify Him. We were brought together for victory. I needed her to get through her season, and she needed me to get through mine. Both helping each other transition, we encouraged one another to stay focused and to push toward excellence. Speaking with her consisted of praying, speaking positive things, and setting goals to break into the next level.

WHEN GOD SPEAKS

There is a boldness that comes when I hear God speak. My confidence rises when I know I listened to exactly what God said. I sought Him, and He answered. Today I heard Him speak clearly. He wanted me to connect with a woman that I barely knew and direct her.

"How would she receive me?" I asked myself as I pondered why God wouldn't direct her Himself. I was tasked to open a door for her and was left speechless when I encountered her. She seemed to have the strongest faith I have ever come across. I listened to her as she shared her heart, wondering what door God would want me to open for her.

I listened intently for God to show me, and without hesitation I became a guide. I wanted her to win, because her win was my win as well!

Spiritual Application of Purpose #12:

Cheer for Your Sisters

- I think this is self-explanatory. You should want everyone to win! Don't be the negative person. Choose to applaud the accolades of each other.
- Take time to find something to be excited about and recognize your sister for it.
- Make it a norm to build up other women and acknowledge their accomplishments.

ONCE IN A LIFETIME

I never would have imagined that when I was asking God for support, He would simultaneously have me help someone. It's reciprocity. God gave me the strength needed to support someone else while I was dealing with the circumstances of my own life. I'm honored. Honored that God heard my cry and helped me to gain insight.

Insight into their world.

"For the LORD giveth wisdom: out of his mouth cometh knowledge and understanding." (Proverbs 2:6 KJV)

I was honored to do so. Representing God, in the form of advice, I was challenged to redefine the term *sisterhood*. Sisterhood means supporting one another, enduring hardships together, and holding each other accountable.

This time my sister passed the test and challenged me.

MAY YOU "LOVE THROUGH" THESE QUESTIONS:

COULD YOU BE HER? The Sister Who Opens Opportunities

- Are you the go-to person for advice among friends and family members?
- Has God shared situations with you in which other people will win?

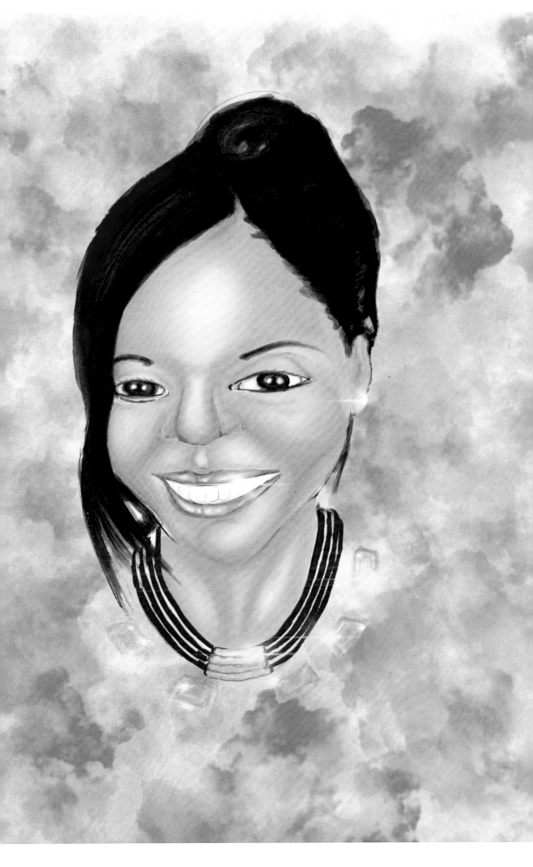

SHE

She sits in a place of silence. An unknown force that creates a significant acknowledgment of emptiness, yet a desire for comfort that she knows.

She thinks she is at a place of discomfort but has no idea the place she resides is a posture that others can see. This is purposeful. For when a light is shown, others can find themselves out of darkness. But light has a burning sensation.

Transfiguration within itself. It can bend itself through rays and make its way in any atmosphere. Does it know the power it holds? Or does the light travel without notice of its shift within the environment?

She is something amazing to behold. Poised in stature. Wise and powerful. She questions her stance while holding onto the Savior, like a life vest. He upholds her so that she can uphold me.

I pray for her protection. For without her constant guidance I am sure my life's direction would have been misled. For there are not many like her.

The drive toward excellence.

The self-assessment against the visions that God has given.

The consistent arrangements for additional supports, when needed.

She understands the importance of order, yet she can see when she is in need of her own covering.

God has placed her in my life for "such a time as this." He knew that our paths would align and one day she would have to testify to me, live her life before me, and give me an example.

Such a great task, but she holds it with grace.

Grace. Sufficient.

Enough to meet the needs of a situation. A sanctification that is unmerited.

Sufficient Grace.

She holds the title well and recognizes that no one but God can help her to transition through this phase. This season where she is being pushed beyond her personal boundaries.

A season of sudden discomfort. Leading to a season of extraordinary blessings.

She is capable of bearing all that God allows her to shoulder.

I observe her forbearances and hold myself accountable to the standard she has set.

She has no idea. Or some idea, that she fights for many.

She fights for me. My well-being. My sanity. My spirituality. My growth in Christ.

Her fight is critical to my health. So when she fights, I fight with her.

In conjunction, we are a team that Satan and his camp fears.

And he should tremble at the thought that God is moving her higher. A force to be reckoned with, she stands as an embodiment of faith, fight, and future.

She is teaching generations to transcend God's power and create awe in the Kingdom.

She is something amazing to behold. Poised in stature. Wise and powerful. She questions her stance while holding onto the Savior like a life vest.

One day, God willing, I will be her.

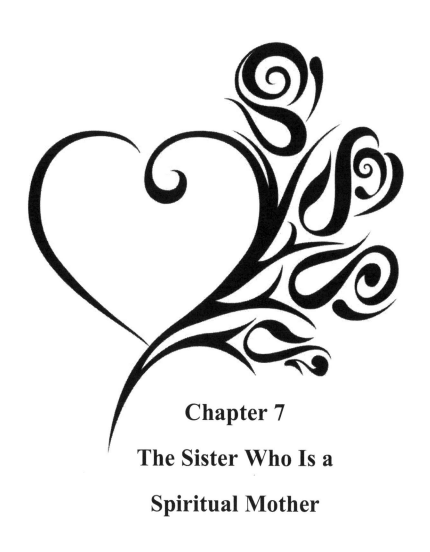

Chapter 7

The Sister Who Is a
Spiritual Mother

BRING LIFE TO ME

LEAD THE WAY

I was called to be a leader. Not that I wanted to be one, but this was the direction that God sent me. I would rather work in the background. Seriously, I'm great at being a worker. But God hasn't spoken that, and He always wins! At a young age, I knew this calling was inevitable. A strange girl with spiritual awareness, linking dreams and visions to words, who would eventually heal others. But this gift would be heavy. "Doesn't everyone's words hold weight?" I asked God, and the answer was complicated.

Remembering the same situations of the women God wanted me to speak to, I was questioning everything. The spirit realm, the natural realm…everything was attached to a question, and this helped me to put things into perspective.

Learning, while God numbered the events in my life that caused heartaches, pain, and betrayal. I wanted God to know I was ready to help my sister get to the Fulfilled Promises. It was a lot to process, but God allowed me to be an example for a reason. God needed me to preach that women should believe, and that God's light can penetrate all situations.

Disgusted at work…Believe God.

Trouble in your marriage…Believe God.

Betrayed by loved ones…Believe God.

Feeling lost and isolated…Believe God.

Although this is often easier said than done, when God is using your life as the example, people begin to revere you as the authority. But I wasn't interested in titles. It seemed that the more titles I had, the greater and more frequent the trials became. My life had become a combination of trials and celebrations. And each one was worth it!

As a leader, I have had my heart broken, my faith tested, and my back against the wall. Every time, God prevailed. He is the only reason why I have walked through fiery traps and came out unscathed.

"Above all, taking the shield of faith, wherewith ye shall be able to quench all the fiery darts of the wicked." (Ephesians 6:16 KJV)

HUMBLE SUBMISSIONS

I'd be the first to admit that I had no idea this task of spiritual guide would be this taxing. The concept of rearing women spiritually requires so much. And because I have been gifted with many daughters in the ministry, I must be mindful of their areas of growth and personality types. Areas of growth will determine how they receive what God places on my heart, and their personality will determine their response. Some will receive what I have to say, others will not.

Have you ever been there?

In a place where you are called by God to speak positivity into someone's life and they will not receive it?

There I was dealing with the major part of this calling...rejection. I was learning that there is always a chance that what God leads me to say, others may take personally. And that was a hard lesson to learn. How can someone who I spend so much time praying for take personally what God gave me? It happens too often!

If this were a movie, it would be entitled *When Spiritual Children Grow Cold*. I say that jokingly, but it is a real thing when people you have loved as your own begin to question your authenticity. I have never guarded myself more than from the betrayal and abandonment, from those who should have been closest to me!

"'Look, I am sending you out as sheep among wolves. So be as shrewd as snakes and harmless as doves.'" (Matthew 10:16 NLT)

Just imagine me covering women who were secretly after me. *Sheep amongst wolves*...God intends for us to be able to step into the territory of wolves and still follow His voice like sheep. I was called to carry the load for other people, but He never said that would be easy. "Continue to cover them: answer their calls, pray for and with them, fast and weep," were my instructions. God was granting me the ability to vouch for souls, even if it came with the title "spiritual mother."

What is a spiritual mother? To be honest, I'm not sure, but I know God has equipped me for it. I have held people accountable, disciplined those who step outside of the established standard, and honored those who ascended into other blessings. He has trusted me to do it.

He trusts me to raise warriors for God's Kingdom, and I believe I'm doing that. God has allowed me to be a part of the spiritual birthing process of so many women. My goals have been to give them the wisdom that God gave me and lead them into a closer relationship with God.

MY HEART CRIES

Becoming a spiritual mother has left me conflicted. Much like natural motherhood, I have been selected to "stand in the gap" spiritually for something that is lacking in these spiritual children. This means that I am usually granted access to things in the spirit that others are not.

My mother used to say things to me like, "I had a feeling," after I told her something. Or, "I already knew," when telling her something that she could not have possibly known. Now this happens to me. God gives me insight for my spiritual sons and daughters and equips me with knowledge and wisdom to know how, and if, I should present it.

Spiritual Application of Purpose #13

When God Gives You Spiritual Insight, Always Ask Him What He Wants You to Do with It

- There are times when God will grant you access to things occurring in the lives of other people. When this happens, ask God what you should do with that information.
- Not everything God gives you should be spoken. Some things you are meant to pray for or against! Have you considered that you might be an intercessor?

Interceding for others requires a specific type of discipline, because no one wants to experience the hardship that comes with this gift. On some nights I lay awake, sit alone, and can feel the spiritual attack occurring. Sometimes, this is the cost of covering someone.

MAY YOU "LOVE THROUGH" THESE QUESTIONS:

COULD YOU BE HER? The Sister Who Is a Spiritual Mother

- Are you considered wise in your circle?
- Can you adequately cover someone, voluntarily, if you knew it would bring you issues?

Section Application: Believe It

RECEPTIVE: able to receive; open and responsive to ideas, impressions, or suggestions.

How does the definition of *receptive* apply to the woman in chapters 6 and 7?

_____
_____
_____
_____
_____

How can you apply the definition of *receptive* to your own life?

_____
_____
_____
_____
_____

THE WOMEN WITHIN

In each chapter, there is a specific type of woman discussed. Describe the woman in chapter 6:

_____
_____
_____

Describe the woman in chapter 7:

_____

_____

_____

What characteristics do these women possess that *enhance* their ability to be used by God?

_____

_____

_____

What characteristics do these women possess that may *hinder* their ability to be used by God?

_____

_____

_____

What are their greatest flaws? What are their greatest strengths?

_____

_____

_____

If you could give advice to these women, what would it be?

Advice for the woman in chapter 6:

_____

_____

_____

_____

Advice   for   the   woman   in   chapter   7:

_____

_____

_____

_____

SCRIPTURAL REFERENCES

Study the following scripture:

"For the LORD giveth wisdom: out of his mouth cometh knowledge and understanding." (Proverbs 2:6 KJV)

What are the key words/terms in this scripture?

_____

_____

_____

_____

How does this scripture apply to the spiritual place that the woman in chapter 6 is in?

_____

_____

_____

_____

Study the following scripture:

"Look, I am sending you out as sheep among wolves. So be as shrewd as snakes and harmless as doves.'" (Matthew 10:16 NLT)

What are the key words/terms in this scripture?

_____

_____

_____

_____

How does this scripture apply to the spiritual place that the woman in chapter 7 is in?

_____

_____

_____

_____

PERSONAL RELEVANCE

Name four ways that you relate to the women in these two chapters.

1. _____
   _____
   _____

2. _____
   _____
   _____

3. _____
   _____
   _____

4. _____
   _____
   _____

LOVING YOU THROUGH IT

Think about who God has placed in your life, as your spiritual mother.

If you belong to a household of faith, this should be a spiritual leader; however, if it is not, it should definitely be someone who is grounded in her own faith.

Who do you consider your spiritual parents?

_____

Share with your spiritual parents your spiritual goals, written in section 2, and write down their observation about your goals.

Make sure to ask the following questions during the conversation:

1. Do you feel this goal is fitting for where I am spiritually?

2. Can you tell I am working on these goals?

3. What areas in my life show evidence that I have a spiritual goal?

4. In what areas is my goal not so evident?

5. What scriptural references could you give me that will help me to focus on these goals?

6. Can you pray for me and my pursuit of these spiritual goals?

Throughout this book, what have you learned about the women who are called to minister to you?

_____

_____

_____

_____

Throughout this book, what have you learned about the woman you were?

_____

_____

_____

_____

Throughout this book, what have you learned about the woman you are becoming?

_____

_____

_____

_____

ROBIN'S REFLECTION

SHE'S NOT

She's not the stereotypical

Created in a godly likeness

She was created by love

Every dip of her eyelash is from a path that was paved

For she is called for His purpose

God alone can ease her pain

She's not the stereotypical

Created in His image

Many waters cannot quench His love for her

It burns like a mighty flame

She's not the stereotypical

SPIRITUAL APPLICATIONS OF PURPOSE

#1: Speak What You Do Not See as if You Already Have It

- Just because it has not come to fruition does not mean it will never happen.
- Keep speaking it! If you are in alignment with God, you can speak things into existence.

#2: If What You Speak Is Not Occurring, Actively Seek God in Prayer to Ensure That What You Are Speaking Is in God's Will

- Prayer and communication with God will allow you access to God's heart concerning what you are seeking.
- Be mindful that God will never give you something that goes against His Word. Example: You are not in God's will if you are asking God to give you someone else's husband. You may be functioning in a spirit of lust or envy, but you are definitely not in God's will.

#3: Take Time to Learn How God Speaks to You

- Take a moment to ask God about one circumstance in your life.
- Pray for God to release all unnecessary thoughts from your mind, especially the ones that are unlike God, and ask God to speak to you about that circumstance.
- Sit, in absolute silence, and write down what you hear in your spirit.

#4: Make Intimate Conversations a Norm

- Analyze how many transparent conversations you have had with sisters.
- Ask yourself the following questions: Can I be vulnerable enough to express my flaws, weaknesses, and secrets to them? Can they do the same?
- Are you sure that your friends will give you a position that aligns with what God says and thinks?

#5: Acknowledge When God Uses Other Forms of Speaking

- God can provide guidance and direction using multiple forms of media.
- When you seek Him, take note of how He speaks to you.
- Does He use the voices of others, sermons, dreams, visions, or songs? Does He allow you to give others the advice you need?
- How God speaks to you is individually packaged for your benefit.

#6: Speak the Truth, Even When It Hurts to Say It

- It may seem easier to hide your thoughts when you are questioning your life, but it will make you feel isolated.
- Expose yourself. Do not be afraid to be who you are…flaws and all!
- Your loved ones, who are living according to God's purpose, will already know you are struggling and will have been praying for your breakthrough. Find out which loved ones are

praying for you, ask God what you can reveal to them and let them hold you accountable for what you can share!

#7: *Ask God for a Strategy*

- Spiritual victory requires God's strategy, so it would behoove you to ask Him for it.
- Be specific in your prayers when asking for strategy. Ask God what you should look for and how He expects you to respond.
- Do not assume that asking for a strategy will give you a quick and automatic win! Some battles are won quickly, and others can span a lifetime.
- The goal is to get to a place where you trust God's lead and follow His word of direction.

#8: *Let Your Heart Break*

- Everyone will give you advice on how to keep yourself together, but who gives you information on how to properly let your heart grieve.
- Tell yourself, "When I am wounded, it is appropriate to be brokenhearted."
- In the moments that you have admitted to heartbreak, know that you need healing. Admit to being brokenhearted, but don't stay there!

#9: *Be an Intentional Listener—You May Have to Share Your Testimony*

- Being a good listener is a burden to bear. It calls for you to listen with your heart and spirit, rather than just your ears. What is their heart expressing?
- If you let them vent, you have made an internal vow to pray over what they speak, uplift their spirit, and push them to grow. You are now responsible for their level of accountability.
- Know that not all listening sessions will be a moment for you to speak, but you should be mindful that your time to share your testimony will come. Be ready!

#10: *Reflect on God's Victories in Your Life*

- What has God brought you through that can be used as a testimony?
- When analyzing victories, what did God reveal about YOU? What characteristics did the battle get rid of that were hindering your personal or spiritual growth?
- It is easy to point out the flaws and growth areas of others, but God wants us to focus on our own!

#11: *Find an Accountability Partner*

- As you mature in Christ, you will need someone who will challenge you to stay consistent with biblical standards.

- Be prepared for your accountability partner to disagree when you are doing something outside the will of God. True accountability partners will check you...in love.

#12: *Cheer for Your Sisters to Win*

- I think this is self-explanatory. You should want everyone to win! Don't be the negative person. Choose to applaud the accolades of each other.
- Take time to find something to be excited about and recognize your sister for it.
- Make it a norm to build up other women and recognize their accomplishments.

#13: *When God Gives You Spiritual Insight, Always Ask Him What He Wants You to Do with It*

- There are times when God will grant you access to things occurring in the lives of other people. When this happens, ask God what you should do with that information.
- Not everything God gives you should be spoken. Some things you are meant to pray for or against! Have you considered that you might be an intercessor?

THE COST OF THIS GIFT

COUNT IT VICTORY

May this book count as a victory. A time where I ended a season of fog and walked into a season of clarity and wins! In the process of writing this book my life changed physically, emotionally, mentally, and spiritually. Many things have ceased to exist as they did at this book's conception, and I am grateful for this! I take note of God's ability to give me the thoughts to write a book for Christian women. Not only was this about a woman's experience, but it was an experience I lived through. I have been every woman in this book. I have been the faithful, the struggling, the untrusting, the mentor, the giver of opportunity, and the spiritual mother to others…these roles do not come without adversity.

For the weight of this book showed itself within my walk, my dreams, and my baggage. I had to be strategic about what I chose to carry during this time. Everything needed to be purposeful and intentional for me to hold on to it. As they say when purposely lifting weights to gain muscle, this book was intentionally "getting my weight up." For I am better as a woman because of the wisdom God has given me to impart. There was not a moment wasted from the circumstances that led me to hear God say, "Name your next book *Loving You Through It*."

I pray this book raised questions about our dedication to the betterment and upbringing of Christian women. I pray, like me, it forced you to examine yourself. I pray it lends itself to workshops and sessions, that will help Christian women discuss openly the topics of healing and deliverance, and how we are responsible for one another. I hope it leads to Bible study and prayer.

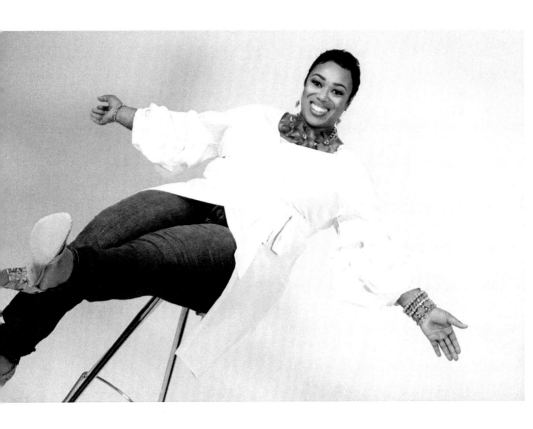

If you would like to contact me for events and speaking engagements, please contact me using the following:

Email: lady.mstredrick@gmail.com

Website: https://ladymithoughtsofmyheart.wordpress.com

About the Author

Misha Stredrick is a speaker, author, and educator, who recently released her first book, "Loving You Through it." She seeks to help people connect their hearts to Christ while making practical steps towards their purpose.

Serving as a middle school principal in Baltimore, Maryland, Misha can be seen functioning from a counselor and disciplinarian to the nurse or mentor. She recognizes that education is a ministry that has no set roles or boundaries, so along the way, she has learned to hold on to God's Promise in Isaiah 43:2-3, "When you go through deep waters, I will be with you. When you go through rivers of difficulty, you will not drown. When you walk through the fire of oppression, you will not be burned up; the flames will not consume you. For I am the Lord, your God, the Holy One of Israel, your Savior."

Misha has Master of Education degrees in Educational Administration, and Curriculum and Instruction, from Bowling Green State University and have been endowed with awards like the Woman of Excellence Award and the OABSE Principal of the Year. She is a contributing writer for the nationally known blog, Daughters of the Deep and the creator of her own blog, entitled: "LadyMi: Thoughts of My Heart," which focuses on Christian living, spiritual growth, Christian relationships, and discipleship.

Misha desires to set the world on fire for living righteously for Christ, while still enjoying spa days, laughing, and the occasional pineapple soda, or two.